LIVING WITH HEPATITIS B

A Survivor's Guide

LIVING WITH HEPATITIS B:

A Survivor's Guide

GREGORY T. EVERSON, M.D., F.A.C.P.

HEDY WEINBERG

HATHERLEIGH PRESS
New York

Hatherleigh Press
5-22 46th Avenue, Suite 200
Long Island City, NY 11101
1-800-528-2550

DISCLAIMER
This book does not give legal or medical advice.
Always consult your lawyer, doctor, and other professionals.
The names of people who contributed anecdotal material have been changed.

The ideas and suggestions contained in this book are not intended as a substitute
for consulting with a physician. All matters regarding your health require medical
supervision.

Library of Congress Cataloging-in-Publication Data
available upon request.

ISBN 1-57826-084-1

All Hatherleigh Press titles are available for special promotions and premiums.
For more information, please contact the manager of our Special Sales department.

Designed by Dede Cummings Designs
Printed in Canada on acid-free paper
10 9 8 7 6 5 4 3 2 1

DEDICATION

To Steve Bingham and Sheree Martin, co-owners and guardians of the Hepatitis B Information and Support List, with thanks for your help and support

To all the people with hepatitis B and their families who shared their stories

To our families, for their understanding and support

With special thanks to Michael Narkewicz, M.D., Medical Director of the Pediatric Liver Center, Marjanne Claassen, R.N., M.S., C.N.S., and Nancy Butler-Simon, M.S., R.N. C.N.S., C.P.N.P., The Children's Hospital in Denver, who contributed their considerable expertise to Chapter 12, "Children with Hepatitis B"

Gregory T. Everson, M.D., F.A.C.P.,
and Hedy Weinberg

CONTENTS

PREFACE

When we were asked to write *Living with Hepatitis B: A Survivor's Guide,* Hedy and I explored the available resources. We found helpful pamphlets, book chapters, and extensive material on the Internet—but no guide dedicated solely to helping you and your family cope with hepatitis B.

Much of the material we reviewed was technical, confusing, and difficult for people to absorb—an understandable situation because hepatitis B is an extremely complex subject. In addition, personal interviews with hepatitis B patients revealed a general lack of knowledge and understanding of this viral infection, of liver disease in general, and of its complications. In short, we found the same situation that prompted us to write our first book, *Living with Hepatitis C: A Survivor's Guide.*

Hepatitis B has a devastating impact on patients and families. It deserves public attention and research dollars. According to the U.S. Centers for Disease Control and Prevention, one out of 20 Americans becomes infected with hepatitis B at some point. Most people recover, but an estimated 1 to 1.25 million remain chronically infected. Globally, the World Health Organization estimates that hepatitis B has infected two billion people; more than 350 million are chronic carriers.

We decided to write a practical guide that takes readers step-by-step through the process of diagnosis and ongoing care. We tried to anticipate questions, translate medical jargon, and reduce the fear of the unknown. Therefore, in addition to medical information, we have also presented overviews of emotional, financial, and nutritional issues that accompany chronic illness.

We hope that this book is useful to you, whether you are newly diagnosed or facing the ongoing challenges of chronic infection. Our primary goals are to present information clearly and to help you cope. Therefore, we asked many people to share their experiences—the funny and hopeful times, as well as the frightening, sad moments.

Throughout the book we emphasize the need for thoughtful wellcontrolled clinical and basic research of hepatitis B. The final chapter speculates on potential breakthroughs in virology, cell biology, and medicine that might lead to a cure of this disease.

One last word: Although *Living with Hepatitis B: A Survivor's Guide* is a detailed reference guide, it does not replace the advice and care of your physician, nor does it give legal advice. Instead, it is designed solely to educate patients and their families about hepatitis B and how it affects their lives. Consult appropriate specialists and always work closely with your doctor when making medical decisions.

FOREWORD

What an excellent gift a copy of *Living with Hepatitis B: A Survivor's Guide* would have been for me in 1981 when I first found out that I had this disease. Now, 20 years later, this book will come in handy as I interact with patients who join our hepatitis B Internet support group. And what a great gift for my family members, my friends, and even my doctors. Beats trying to explain the complexities of HBV myself!

The "newbies" to our on-line support group come to us with the same feelings of fear and confusion that I remember all too well. Especially the confusion. I don't think there's a disease more bewildering than HBV for both patients and doctors.

Gregory T. Everson, M.D., a noted hepatologist, and Hedy Weinberg, a writer and hepatitis patient, make an ideal writing team. They manage to translate complicated medical terminology and to untangle the most common problems facing those of us infected or affected by HBV. The authors have tackled some particularly difficult, but relevant, topics with their chapters on finance, liver transplants, liver cancer, co-infection, and pediatric HBV.

Because it is difficult-to-impossible to find a local, live HBV support group, I appreciate the support-group feeling of this patient's guide. When I was first diagnosed, I wanted to find others who were going through the same things that I was going through. Here, in this book, the reader will find many new friends speaking out on every possible subject related to hepatitis B. The authors have included the voices of many HBV survivors. Some of the patient quotes made me smile, and some gave me a jolt as I identified and remembered my own experiences.

I also like the optimistic tone of *Living with Hepatitis B: A Survivor's Guide*. The majority of us chronic HBV patients will survive the disease in the sense that we won't die from it, but few of us are apt to conquer and clear the virus completely. So the challenge is learning to live with the disease while, at the same time, not letting ourselves become the disease. The authors suggest positive ways to maintain a high quality of life. They reassure us that we can still experience major victories along the way, some physical and some psychological. We begin to understand that living with HBV is a victory in itself.

Overall, I'm just grateful that this book was written. It is unique and fills an important niche—an entire book specifically addressing the issues of HBV patients. Sometimes those of us with HBV feel frustrated when other less common or less serious diseases seem to get more attention and publicity. But one of the most encouraging things that we learn from reading the final chapter, appropriately subtitled "Hope for the Future," is that we aren't being ignored by scientists and that there is a surprising amount of research going on.

With the publication of *Living with Hepatitis B: A Survivor's Guide*, we who deal every day with the challenges of hepatitis B can truly say that we are not alone.

Steve Bingham
Co-listowner, Hepatitis B Information and Support List

ACKNOWLEDGMENTS

With appreciation and gratitude to the hard-working, dedicated members of the Liver Team at the University of Colorado Health Sciences Center: Thomas Trouillot, M.D.; James Trotter, M.D.; Marcelo Kugelmas, M.D.; Greg Fitz, M.D.; Igal Kam, M.D., Chief of Division of Transplant Surgery; Michael Wachs, M.D.; Thomas Bak, M.D.; Susan Mandell, M.D.; Thomas Beresford, M.D.; Barbara Fey, R.N., M.S.N., Hepatology Nurse; Cathy Ray, R.N., B.S.N., M.A., Hepatology Nurse; Jim Epp, R.N., B.S.N., Hepatology Nurse; Megan Dyer, Lori Carrillo, Ariana Wallack, Administrative Assistants; Medical Assistants Justin Skilbred, M.A.; Chris Tomasi, C.M.A.; Jennifer DeSanto, R.N., Research Coordinator; Melissa Douglass, R.N., B.S.N., Research Coordinator; Carol McKinley, R.N., Research Coordinator; Radene Showalter, Laboratory Researcher; Sue Sellissen, P.R.A.; Shannon Lauritski; Tracy Steinberg, R.N., M.S., C.C.T.C.; Tim Brackett, R.N.; Mary McClure, R.N.; Michael Talamantes, M.S.S.W., L.C.S.W.

Also from the University of Colorado Health Sciences Center, we thank Robert M. House, M.D., Associate Professor, Director, Residency Training, Department of Psychiatry; Patrick M. Klem, PharmD., B.C.P.S., Hannis W. Thompson, M.D., Associate Medical Director, Bonfils Blood Center, Director of Transfusion Medicine, University of Colorado Medical School; Steven C. Johnson, M.D., Associate Professor of Medicine, Director of the University Hospital HIV/AIDS Clinical Program; Mary Bessesen, M.D., Infectious Disease Clinic, VA Medical Center; Fabi Imo, Coordinator, Transplant Financial Services; Patty Polsky, M.B.A., Manager, Registration and Financial Services; Rev. Julie Swaney, University Hospital Chaplain.

Dr. Everson wishes to further acknowledge the support of the staff at University Hospital and the University of Colorado Health Sciences Center in the care and management of patients with hepatitis B.

From The Children's Hospital Pediatric Liver Center, we thank Michael Narkewicz, M.D., Section of Pediatric Gastroenterology, Hepatology and Nutrition, Hewit/Andrews Chair in Pediatric Liver Disease, and Medical Director of the Pediatric Liver Center, who reviewed Chapter 12 and gave generously of his time and practical advice, and Ronald Sokol, M.D., Professor of Pediatrics, Director of the Pediatric General Clinical Research Center; Marjanne Claassen, R.N., M.S., C.N.S., Clinical Nurse Specialist, Pediatric Liver Center Coordinator, and Nancy Butler-Simon, M.S., R.N., C.N.S., C.P.N.P., Advanced Practice Nurse, Pediatric General Clinical Research Center, who added advice and practical help for parents; and the Pediatric Transplant Team, including Fritz Karrer, M.D.

We thank Steve Potter, Public Affairs Specialist, Denver Social Security, for reviewing our information on Social Security issues; and Meredith Pate-Willig, M.S.W., L.C.S.W., for her help with the chapter on the emotional challenges of chronic illness.

In addition, we thank all the members of the Hepatitis B Information and Support List. They helped identify the problems, fears, and triumphs of people with hepatitis B and cheered us on through the writing process. We are most grateful to Steve Bingham and Sheree Martin, co-owners of the listserv, who give so much of themselves every day. They encouraged and supported us all the way. Special mention and kudos go to their "hepper-helpers," Jack Leonard and Doug Martin.

We'd also like to thank the following people for their help and for their contributions to the welfare of people with hepatitis B: Molli Conti, Associate Director, Hepatitis B Foundation; Alan P. Brownstein, President and CEO, American Liver Foundation; Thelma King Thiel, Chair and CEO, Hepatitis Foundation International; and Trish Parnell, Director, Parents of Kids with Infectious Diseases.

Most important of all, we are grateful to all the patients and their families who opened their hearts and shared their stories.

1

WHAT IS HEPATITIS B?

An Introduction

Twelve years ago, I noticed I was feeling weak, but I figured it was due to a major move I was making from California. The fatigue persisted. Weekends were spent in bed catching up on the sleep I wasn't getting during the week. After the move, I went in for a complete medical checkup. The doctor called at 10 o'clock that night and told me I tested positive for hepatitis B. "It's gone chronic," he said. "I want to see you right away."

I didn't think much of it except that doctors don't usually call at that hour. I told him I had no idea what he was talking about. I didn't feel alarmed because I didn't know anything about hepatitis B.

John

IF YOU'VE JUST been told you have hepatitis B, you may feel uncertain and confused. A diagnosis of liver disease raises a lot of questions: "What is hepatitis B? How did I get infected? Can I infect others? Is there treatment? If I tell them at work, will they fire me?"

Hepatitis B (HBV) is a viral infection that causes inflammation, injury, and ultimately scarring of the liver (cirrhosis). That sounds frightening, but remember: you are not alone. Estimates show that more than a million Americans are chronically infected with hepatitis B. Each year 140,000 to 320,000 people contract the virus, but most fight off the infection.

Once people are infected with hepatitis B, outcomes vary (see Figure 1A). Ninety to 95 percent of adults clear the virus and gain lifelong immunity to hepatitis B, but five to 10 percent do not clear hepatitis B and remain chronically infected. Some of these chronically infected patients have abnormal liver tests and liver biopsies, reflecting ongoing liver damage. We say that they have chronic hepatitis B.

What about the chronically infected patients who have normal liver tests and liver biopsies? These patients typically have little or no liver damage but can pass the infection to others. We call them "chronic carriers." Carriers have active viral infection but lack liver damage and are otherwise healthy. However, some carriers experience flares of hepatitis, and carriers who became infected at birth from their mothers are at risk of developing liver cancer (see Figure 1B).

Although chronic hepatitis B is a serious problem, the infection usually progresses slowly over years or decades. Chronic hepatitis B can

FIGURE 1A. CONSEQUENCES OF HEPATITIS B (HBV) INFECTION.

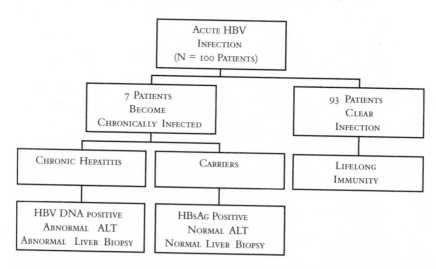

LEGEND 1A: This figure shows the consequences of infection with hepatitis B. The vast majority of patients infected with hepatitis B clear the infection and develop lifelong immunity. Five to 10% develop chronic infection. Carriers have ongoing viral infection (positive HBsAg) but lack evidence of liver injury. Patients with chronic hepatitis have viral infection (positive HBV DNA), liver injury with elevated liver enzymes (ALT), and damage on biopsy.

FIGURE IB. POSSIBLE OUTCOMES IN PATIENTS WITH CHRONIC HEPATITIS B INFECTION.

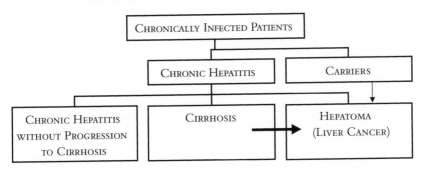

LEGEND IB: Chronically infected patients are at risk for cirrhosis and liver cancer. Inflammation and damage to the liver results in formation of scar tissue (fibrosis) that ultimately can progress to cirrhosis. Cirrhosis of the liver impairs function and leads to clinical consequences (see Chapter 4). The major risk for liver cancer is in patients with chronic hepatitis and cirrhosis (approximately 2%/yr). Carriers, who lack liver injury, are still at risk for liver cancer, especially if they have had the infection for more than 20 years.

be dangerous if it damages your liver to the point of cirrhosis. In fact, about 4,000 to 5,000 Americans die from liver disease or liver cancer due to hepatitis B every year. As you can see from the mortality figures, however, it's far more likely that you will have to learn to *live* with the virus until scientists find a cure. That's what this book is about: how to live with and survive hepatitis B.

A Word of Caution: Information in this book does not substitute for the advice of your physician. If you have hepatitis B, you should be under a doctor's care.

In this chapter we'll discuss some basic facts and statistics about hepatitis B, the history and discovery of the hepatitis B virus and vaccines, and information about viruses and other forms of viral hepatitis. Here are the topics we'll cover:

- You Are Not Alone
- Understanding Hepatitis B
  What Is Hepatitis?
  What Is a Virus?

What Is the Hepatitis B Virus (HBV)?
- A Public Health Problem
- The Discovery of Hepatitis B
    - *Hepatitis B Vaccines*
- The Hepatitis Viral Alphabet
    - *Hepatitis A*
    - *Hepatitis B*
    - *Hepatitis C*
    - *Hepatitis D*
    - *Hepatitis E*
    - *Hepatitis ?F, X, TTV, SEN?*
    - *Hepatitis G*
- Hepatitis B: How Close Is a Cure?

You Are Not Alone

If you or someone you love has hepatitis B, know that you're not alone. According to the U.S. Centers for Disease Control and Prevention (CDC), one out of 20 Americans will become infected with hepatitis B at some time in their lives. They may show no symptoms at all or suffer an acute attack with flu-like symptoms of fatigue; mild fever; vomiting or diarrhea; loss of appetite; nausea; muscle, joint, and stomach pain; and, in some cases, jaundice (yellowing of the eyes and skin). Most people recover, but the CDC estimates that 1 to 1.25 million—one out of every 200 Americans—remain chronically infected.

Globally, hepatitis B is a severe problem. The World Health Organization estimates that hepatitis B has infected two billion people worldwide. More than *350 million* are chronic carriers of the virus. The highest rates of hepatitis B occur in the developing world: sub-Saharan Africa, most of Asia and the Pacific rim, the Amazon, the southern parts of Eastern and Central Europe, portions of the Middle East, and the Indian subcontinent (see Figure 1C).

In Northern Europe and North America, infection rates are lower, and less than 1 percent are chronic carriers. It's hard to relate to these numbers and percentages, so let's make the statistics more real. The number of people in the United States with hepatitis B is more than the number of people with HIV/AIDS, triple that of Parkinson's, and five times the number of Americans with multiple sclerosis.

In my state of Colorado, with its population of approximately 4 million, I estimate that 20,000 persons are chronically infected with hepati-

FIGURE IC. WORLDWIDE DISTRIBUTION OF HEPATITIS B

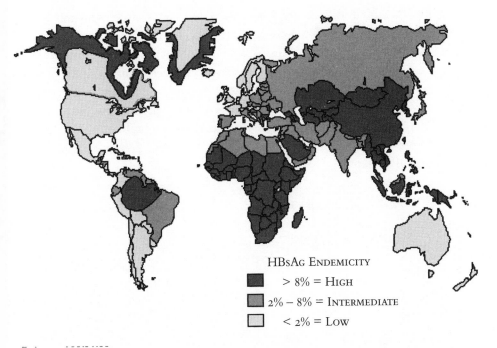

HBsAg Endemicity
> 8% = High
2% – 8% = Intermediate
< 2% = Low

LEGEND IC: Geographic Pattern of Hepatitis B Prevalence, 1997. This map shows the worldwide distribution of hepatitis B. High prevalence populations are located predominantly in sub-Saharan Africa, Central and Southeast Asia, the Amazon region of South America, and the native populations of Alaska, Canada and Greenland [World Health Organization (WHO)].

tis B. Data from the Colorado Department of Health supports this figure. From 1990 through June 2000, 7,290 cases of chronic hepatitis B were reported. Yet for the majority of patients, chronic hepatitis B presents no symptoms. Therefore, patients do not seek medical attention or treatment, and most cases of chronic hepatitis B go undetected. If we realistically assume that only one-third of the cases in Colorado were reported, there are 21, 870 cases in the state. Therefore, the calculated prevalence is that one out of every 200 Coloradans has chronic hepatitis B—identical to the national prevalence.

Although the public doesn't realize it, chronic hepatitis B is a common, serious, and significant infectious disease in my state and in the

United States. But numbers and statistics don't tell the whole story. When you're diagnosed with hepatitis B, you may feel as alone as you can possibly feel. It's as if an invisible fence has gone up between you and all the other people who don't have hepatitis. You have an infectious illness; they don't. You're worried about yourself, and you're worried about the people you love. You're angry. Perhaps you even feel ashamed.

Hepatitis puts a heavy strain on relationships. Close friends, who used to hug and kiss you, may become distant or even pull away. People don't tell their bosses and co-workers because they might lose their jobs. Lovers are afraid to touch one another. Mothers and fathers hesitate to cook for their families.

> *I didn't keep anything back. No secrets. I told everyone I had hepatitis B. I was so naïve.*
>
> *Once, my friends were gathering names to help make food for a funeral. I volunteered to bake a pie, and the woman in charge said, "Maybe you could buy the pie." I knew right away what she was implying. So I bought a pie.*
>
> *Nora*

A healthy dose of facts about hepatitis B helps people deal with their fears. You can touch people; you can cook for them. Hepatitis B is not spread by casual contact. Tell your family, friends, neighbors, and bosses that to get infected, their skin would have to be punctured with contaminated blood or saliva. The hepatitis B virus is found in blood, semen, and vaginal secretions. People get it from unprotected sex with an infected person, shared drug needles, tattoos, body-piercing, borrowed razors, and close personal contact with infected members of the household.

> *We adopted a child from Poland twelve years ago. He seemed healthy. We knew nothing about hepatitis, and our pediatrician didn't think of it. We were so ignorant.*
>
> *Our son had a genetic disorder, delayed blood clotting. He used to hurt himself a lot, like any other kid, but of course he didn't clot well and bled a lot. So if he skinned his knee or something, I would do the motherly thing and kiss the hurt, and clean up the blood.*

About three years after the adoption, I started to get sick all the time. I went through 12 to 13 prescriptions for antibiotics in one year. Then my blood tests started to show elevated liver enzymes. I had hepatitis B.

We tested the family. Everyone else had antibodies, but David had the virus. I got hepatitis B from my own son.

Janice

People at risk are those exposed to blood or body fluids of an infected person. The list includes health care workers; those who live or work in health care facilities or prisons; police and fire personnel; babies born to mothers with hepatitis B; hemophiliacs or patients on hemodialysis; travelers to or immigrants from countries where hepatitis B is prevalent; people who have unprotected sex with a carrier or chronically infected person; people who live in a household with an infected person; intravenous drug users; and persons who are bitten by someone whose saliva contains the virus. If you received a blood transfusion in the United States after 1975, you have almost no risk of contracting hepatitis B in this way.

But many people have no idea how they became infected. According to the American Liver Foundation (ALF), 30 to 40 percent don't know when or how they came into contact with contaminated blood or body fluids.

Understanding Hepatitis B

To understand hepatitis B, it helps to define three terms:

- hepatitis
- virus
- hepatitis B virus or HBV

What Is Hepatitis? Hepatitis simply means inflammation of the liver. Many injurious agents can cause hepatitis, including alcohol, medications, drugs, toxins, or viruses.

Unfortunately, the public hears so many stories of celebrities who injured their livers with substance abuse that they tend to lump all forms of liver disease together. As anyone with hepatitis B can tell you, it's not uncommon (although extremely unfair) to be labeled an alcoholic, even if you've never taken a drink.

I had what's called a "variceal bleed." I was bleeding from my throat and got 13 units of blood. When I woke up in the hospital, they kept asking me if I was an alcoholic.

"Are you sure you don't need a drink every morning when you get up?" they asked me. It was right before Christmas, and they said that lots of heavy drinkers showed up in the emergency room with the same problem. I remember feeling offended.

After eight days, the tests came back. It was a relief to hear that I had hepatitis B, because they finally stopped questioning me about alcohol.

Janet

What Is a Virus? The name virus evokes fear in people, fear of the unknown. Viruses are not visible to the human eye or by standard microscopy; you need an electron microscope to see them. During the past 30 years, scientists have discovered hepatitis viruses A through G. Despite their small size, viruses carry genetic material with enough punch to injure our organs and bodies and even cause death.

Viruses are as old as humankind—possibly older. Archeologists have unearthed an Egyptian mummy that bears pockmarks, evidence of the smallpox virus thousands of years ago. Among other diseases, viruses cause polio, mononucleosis, rabies, herpes, yellow fever, influenza, measles, rubella, chicken pox, mumps, the common cold—and new plagues, such as Ebola and AIDS.

"A virus," said Nobel Laureate Sir Peter Medawar, "is a piece of bad news wrapped in protein."[1] And that about sums it up. A virus contains a center of nucleic acid (the viral genes) surrounded by a protein coat.

When a virus's coat attaches to a cell in the body, the virus's genes enter the cell. They order the cell to stop its own work and to make more viruses instead. In time, the virus multiplies to infect other cells.

Alerted to danger, the body's immune system sends out antibodies to stick to the invading virus and neutralize it. Viruses, however, are able to change and mutate to evade these antibodies.

What Is the Hepatitis B Virus (HBV)? Hepatitis B is a partially double-stranded deoxyribonucleic acid (DNA) virus and a member of the hepadnavirus family. Other members of this family include the duck hepatitis virus and woodchuck hepatitis virus.

What is DNA? DNA lives in the center of each cell in your body in 46 threadlike chromosomes (23 pairs) that contain the genes that make you a unique human being. DNA makes the proteins that create cells. If you took the DNA from just one of your cells and stretched it out, it would measure about six feet!

The hepatitis B virus has its own DNA and is very complex. When it gets into your liver cells, it takes on complicated coiled and uncoiled forms and even invades your own liver cells' DNA.

To add to the complexity, scientists have recently discovered multiple genetic forms (genotypes) of hepatitis B. Obviously, a detailed description of hepatitis B molecular and cell biology is well beyond the scope of this book. Nonetheless, certain basic information is essential to improve your understanding of this infection and the tests used to detect the virus.

The blood test most commonly used to detect hepatitis B is the hepatitis B surface antigen (HBsAg). This surface antigen is a protein made by a specific gene located in the viral DNA and is the key component of the virus coat. Positive surface antigen is an indication that a patient is infected with hepatitis B.

Another common test is the hepatitis B surface antibody (HBsAb). This is an antibody made by a person who has been infected and cleared hepatitis B; it does not measure the virus, just the person's response to the infection. Positive surface antibody is an indication that a patient has been exposed to surface antigen either by infection with hepatitis B or after vaccination with hepatitis B vaccine.

Other tests indicate that the virus is actively reproducing itself, or replicating. These tests include the hepatitis B e antigen (HBeAg) and the hepatitis B viral DNA count (HBV DNA) and are used primarily during a course of antiviral treatment to monitor effectiveness (see Chapter 2).

A Public Health Problem

Hepatitis B is a serious but underappreciated public health problem. The virus is 50 to 100 times more infectious than HIV, the virus that causes AIDS. Although the Federal Food and Drug Administration (FDA) approved a vaccine in 1981, the majority of the U.S. population has not received the series of three doses and is therefore still at risk. Furthermore, immigration from areas with a high prevalence of hepatitis B constantly increases the pool of individuals with the virus in this country.

In addition, an estimated 40 percent of patients with chronic hepatitis B and nearly all surface-antigen carriers have no signs or symptoms. Therefore, the majority of patients is unaware of infection and may unknowingly spread the virus. Liver disease is usually a silent illness, and people may not have severe symptoms until the end stages—a process that, if it occurs, may take decades.

Some chronically ill patients have milder inflammation and do not progress to cirrhosis, while others endure severe liver inflammation and progress to cirrhosis. Liver cancer (hepatocellular carcinoma or hepatoma) may complicate chronic infection, especially in patients with underlying cirrhosis.

The frustrating problem is that we can't predict outcomes for individual patients with exact precision. The virus can lurk in the body for years and years like a time bomb, silently injuring your liver and setting the stage for complications from liver disease.

> *I'm a doctor so one day when I rubbed my abdomen, I noticed that my liver was enlarged. I thought my emphysema was getting worse and pushing my liver down.*
>
> *I went in for a physical checkup, and the doctor ordered tests. My ALT was 600, and my SGOT was 500, but I was in total denial. I felt fine. I thought maybe I just needed medicine for a bum knee.*
>
> *My biopsy showed a mess! The normal lobular pattern was gone. I had cirrhosis. Crap. Everyone felt quite dismal about it.*
>
> *Martin*

The Discovery of Hepatitis B

Since ancient times, people have known about hepatitis and the jaundice that sometimes accompanies the infection. They thought unsanitary conditions caused the illness, particularly because many epidemics occurred in wartime. Then, during World War II, a new yellow fever vaccine was administered to army recruits. Although no one knew it, the vaccine was contaminated with blood serum infected with hepatitis viruses. The vaccine protected against yellow fever but gave many soldiers jaundice. Researchers finally linked hepatitis to blood exposure.

In the mid-1950s and 1960s Dr. Saul Krugman investigated forms of hepatitis that were endemic (occurring nearly universally due to natural exposures) in the Willowbrook State School for retarded children in Staten Island, New York. His studies, although controversial from the standpoint of informed consent and experimentation on human subjects, showed that the outbreaks of hepatitis at the school were caused by two separate strains of virus. One had a short incubation period, was transmitted primarily by fecal-oral contamination, did not enter a chronically infected stage, and was later determined to be hepatitis A. The other had a longer incubation period, was transmitted primarily by contact with contaminated blood, did enter a chronic stage in a small proportion of patients, and was later determined to be hepatitis B.

During the 1960s, Dr. Baruch Blumberg was researching genetic differences by examining the blood of people around the world who had received transfusions. When people receive blood, they produce antibodies (special types of proteins that defend against foreign proteins). Dr. Blumberg discovered antibodies in the blood of a patient with hemophilia living in New York that reacted with the blood of an Australian aborigine. Therefore, a foreign protein, called an antigen, was present in the aborigine's blood and was bound to, or reacted with, a specific antibody in the New York hemophiliac's blood. He named the antigen after Australia, calling it the Australian or Au antigen.

In 1966, a teenager named James Bair, who had previously tested negative for the Au antigen in Dr. Blumberg's study, fell ill with hepatitis and subsequently became positive for Au antigen when retested. The connection was finally made between the Au antigen and hepatitis. That same year, one of Dr. Blumberg's technicians fell ill and became the first person diagnosed with hepatitis B using the Au antigen test.

Further research determined that the Australia antigen was the surface antigen of hepatitis B. The first tests for hepatitis B, developed in 1971, were relatively insensitive. In 1972 the Food and Drug Administration (FDA) mandated testing of donated blood, and the following year the American Association of Blood Banks began to require testing for the surface antigen in order to screen blood donations. In 1975 highly sensitive and specific radioimmunoassays and enzyme immunoassays were introduced.

Today the nation's blood supply is relatively safe. The current average risk of getting hepatitis B from a single unit of transfused blood is one in 63,000. If you received a transfusion prior to 1975, however, you may have contracted the virus in this way.

A great big snowstorm came up that week. The supervisor told me to keep the construction crew working. Two to three feet of snow covered the ground, including a large hole—three feet wide and three feet deep. I was looking up at the fence and fell in that hole.

During the surgery to remove my top rib, the doctor nicked an artery. They checked my blood pressure, and I didn't have any. That artery bled down all inside my stomach cavity. They told me the operating room was covered in blood.

Everybody in my church gave blood. I got 44 units! When I woke up three days later, the doctor said, "You have hepatitis and it's type B. We're going to have to check you for the rest of your life." That was almost 30 years ago. I was just happy to be alive.

Barry

Dr. Blumberg received a Nobel Prize for Medicine in 1976. Extraordinary gains in basic and clinical research and in the understanding of hepatitis B rapidly followed this milestone. Within five years, the prevention of hepatitis B was in sight when the Federal Drug Administration approved the first hepatitis B vaccine. In 1986, scientists succeeded in growing the virus in a test tube, and today the virus has been completely sequenced, all the functional genetic elements are known, and all relevant viral proteins have been identified.

Hepatitis B Vaccines. Dr. Blumberg and Dr. Irving Millman invented the first vaccine for hepatitis B in 1969. The vaccine was commercially developed during the 1970s. Since 1982, safe and effective hepatitis B vaccines have been available and have provided prolonged, perhaps life-long, protection.

The first vaccines were plasma–derived vaccines of purified surface antigen. They were prepared from human plasma obtained from patients chronically infected with hepatitis B. These vaccines proved to be safe and effective, but fear of transmission of other known (HIV) or unknown viruses led to rapid development of purified vaccines prepared by recombinant DNA technology. The currently available vaccines, Engerix B® and Recombivax® are prepared in this way.

More than a billion doses of hepatitis B vaccine have been administered across the globe, saving countless lives. Unfortunately, developing countries find it hard to afford the cost. Of course, the vaccine will not cure someone who is already infected, but the hepatitis B vaccine is a tremendous advance in health care. In fact, scientists call it the first vaccine against cancer (because liver cancer is a complication of advanced hepatitis B) and the first vaccine against a sexually transmitted disease.

The Hepatitis Viral Alphabet

When you tell someone you have hepatitis B, you usually end up fielding a lot of questions: "How do you get hepatitis B? Can I catch it from you? From dirty food?" It helps to know the facts about the hepatitis alphabet—from A to G.

As you now know, hepatitis means inflammation of the liver. Although drugs, toxins, and many other exposures also can inflame the liver, the most common cause of hepatitis is viral. Hepatitis viruses primarily attack the liver, while other viruses (such as the herpes or mononucleosis viruses) injure the liver as part of a generalized infection.

We know at least six, and possibly seven, distinct hepatitis viruses, identified by the letters A through G. Blood tests distinguish and diagnose the different forms, but the public tends to lump them all together.

Hepatitis A. Outbreaks of this virus occur because of poor hygiene—a contaminated water supply or, for example, inadequate hand washing in a day-care facility. Hepatitis A, excreted in feces, is the most common cause of food or waterborne epidemic hepatitis. Areas of high prevalence include Mexico, Central America, sub-Saharan Africa, Southeast Asia, and the Middle East.

People who contract hepatitis A typically develop flu-like symptoms within 10 to 40 days of exposure (the acute stage). They experience low-grade fever, muscle aches, joint aches, headache, malaise, anorexia, and mild abdominal pain. Often, but not always, these symptoms are rapidly followed by jaundice, a yellowing of the whites of the eyes and skin. In the vast majority of cases, the patient recovers completely with lifelong immunity against re-infection.

Hepatitis A never persists after the acute infection, so people don't develop chronic hepatitis, cirrhosis, or liver cancer. Rarely, in approximately one out of 1,000 cases, does the patient have severe acute hepatitis leading to liver failure and urgent need for transplantation. A vaccine is available for hepatitis A.

Hepatitis B. Hepatitis B spreads through blood inoculation: transfusions of blood or blood products, intravenous illicit drug use, hemodialysis, cardiac bypass surgery, or accidental needle-stick. It also spreads readily by sexual contact, both heterosexual and homosexual, close personal contact, and can easily be transmitted from mother to infant at delivery.

Two years ago, I went to the doctor for back pain. My blood counts had been fluctuating drastically for a while so the doctor drew blood. They checked for hepatitis, and the test came back positive for hepatitis B.

I wasn't surprised. My mother and two aunts died of hepatitis B. I think I got it from my mother at birth. After my mom died, I was thinking about having myself checked, but I never did.

Matt

Ninety to 95 percent of adults infected with hepatitis B clear the infection and maintain lifelong immunity. Rarely, a patient may develop liver failure from severe acute hepatitis B. The remaining 5 to 10 percent do not clear the virus. They become carriers or develop chronic hepatitis and risk progression to cirrhosis or liver cancer.

Untreated newborns who acquire hepatitis B from their mothers often develop lifelong infection. The good news is that treating the newborn with HBIG (hepatitis B immune globulin) and hepatitis B vaccine immediately after delivery prevents transmission in more than 95 percent of cases.

People with acute hepatitis B have the same symptoms as people with any other form of acute hepatitis. Chronic sufferers may not have symptoms or may complain of chronic fatigue, malaise, poor energy, and episodic jaundice.

Current FDA-approved medical therapies for chronic hepatitis B are interferon alfa-2b (INTRON® A, Schering-Plough) and lamivudine (EPIVIR-HBV®, Glaxo Wellcome). Other potentially effective antiviral agents under study include ganciclovir, lobucavir, adefovir dipivoxil, thymosin-alpha1, and famciclovir.

Liver transplantation for hepatitis B is highly effective with low rates of recurrence. Patients who need transplants for severe acute hepatitis seldom, if ever, develop hepatitis B in the transplanted liver. The virus may recur in transplants performed for chronic liver disease, but use of lamivudine and long-term immune globulin therapy after the transplantation reduces that risk.

Hepatitis C. An estimated 3.9 million Americans have hepatitis C. It is the most prevalent form of chronic hepatitis in the United States, accounting for 20 to 25 percent of all hepatitis cases. We now believe that it becomes chronic in 75 to 85 percent of infected people.

The infection is transmitted by blood, like hepatitis B. However, unlike hepatitis B, it seems to be poorly transmitted by sexual contact and is infrequently passed (6 percent) from an otherwise healthy mother to her newborn.

Most infected people may not be aware that they had a past episode of acute hepatitis. In general, symptoms of acute hepatitis C are mild and liver enzyme elevations in the blood are modest. Two chronically infected patients may have identical symptoms and liver enzyme tests but very different results from a biopsy—from mild, benign histology (the study of the liver tissue under the microscope) to advanced injury with cirrhosis.

Patients may be candidates for interferon therapy or the combination of interferon plus ribavirin. New agents currently under investigation or development include long-acting (pegylated) interferons, ribozymes, and protease inhibitors.

Today, hepatitis C is the leading indication for liver transplantation. Twenty to 40 percent of patients on liver transplant waiting lists have hepatitis C. The virus recurs in the transplanted liver, and treatment may be necessary.

Hepatitis D. Hepatitis D, or delta hepatitis, is an incomplete virus that requires the presence of hepatitis B in order to complete its life cycle. For this reason, delta is typically found only in patients who have hepatitis B. Most patients with chronic hepatitis B, however, are not co-infected with hepatitis D.

Risk factors are the same as for hepatitis B. Hepatitis B patients co-infected with delta have a greater chance of developing fulminant hepatitis (a sudden, severe attack), more severe chronic active hepatitis, and an increased rate of progression to cirrhosis. The virus does not seem to have a major effect on hepatitis B patients' response to interferon therapy or on their survival or on the recurrence of hepatitis B after a liver transplant.

Hepatitis E. Symptoms are the same as hepatitis A, but cases in the United States appear to be imports from Central America, Mexico, and the Indian subcontinent of Asia. In most instances, patients don't become chronic carriers, and the virus is not associated with hepatocellular cancer.

Currently no vaccine or specific medical therapy exists. If acquired during pregnancy, hepatitis E has been associated with high rates of maternal and fetal mortality. The Centers for Disease Control and Prevention in Atlanta, Georgia, offer testing.

Hepatitis ?F, X, TTV, SEN? Some patients with viral hepatitis lack evidence for infection with hepatitis A through E. Studies of these patients have uncovered potential new hepatitis viruses. The story is not fully in on these viruses. Early reports have suggested that they may cause sporadic hepatitis, chronic hepatitis, and perhaps progression to liver failure.

Hepatitis G. We're learning more about this newly discovered virus, which is transmitted in the same way as hepatitis C. Hepatitis C and hepatitis G are in the same family of viruses, and hepatitis G is comprised of at least four main subtypes. But we don't know whether hepatitis G causes clinically significant liver disease.

Reports indicate that as many as 20 percent of hepatitis C patients may also be infected with hepatitis G. However, there's no evidence that hepatitis G independently causes chronic progressive hepatitis.

Hepatitis B: How Close Is a Cure?

The global prevention for hepatitis B exists—an effective vaccine to eradicate the disease. Unfortunately, the cost of the vaccine has prohibited its worldwide use. Vaccination programs in the United States, aimed at children, should eventually eliminate the disease in our population. However, cases from regions of the world with a high prevalence of hepatitis B will continue to immigrate into the U.S. and maintain the pool of infected persons. It is gratifying to see countries, such as China with the aid of the World Health Organization, begin to allocate resources to vaccination programs in an attempt to deal with the worldwide problem of hepatitis B.

How close is a cure? Current therapies for patients with chronic hepatitis B are only partially effective. The best results are obtained with interferon, but this treatment is expensive and associated with many adverse side effects. Lamivudine is highly effective in suppressing hepatitis B and has few side effects, but only a small proportion sustain the antiviral effect after treatment is discontinued and long-term use is associated with the emergence of mutant forms of hepatitis B that are resistant to lamivudine.

New treatments currently under investigation include specialized vaccines, additional antivirals such as adefovir and ribavirin, immunotherapy, and ribozymes. Although the majority of the 1.25 million U.S. patients will not respond to current treatments, future treatments offer the hope for cure of the disease.

As a doctor, I'm excited when a patient conquers and clears the hepatitis B virus. Those who fail to clear the virus still have other victories along the way. Any illness, especially a chronic one, tests a person's limits. My hope is that the following chapters will help you learn more about hepatitis B and make you more comfortable with your choices and challenges from day to day.

The beginning of wisdom is to call things by their right names.

Chinese proverb

Reference
1 Peter Radetsky, *The Invisible Invaders: Viruses and the Scientists Who Pursue Them* (Boston: Little Brown and Co., 1994) p. 8.

2

WHEN YOU HAVE HEPATITIS B

Understanding the Diagnosis: Blood Tests and Biopsies

I got home from a family reunion exhausted. When I woke up Monday morning, I looked in the mirror. My skin and the whites of my eyes were yellow, jaundiced! I knew I was sick.

The doctor did blood tests for all kinds of hepatitis. I had to contact all the members of my family because at first we didn't know if it was hepatitis A. It turned out to be hepatitis all right, but it was hepatitis B.

Jim

W HEN I TELL my patients their blood tests show that they have hepatitis B, some are shocked. Others, however, can recall a prior attack of hepatitis, an illness with jaundice, or a risk factor. All of us, when we hear upsetting news, have the same reaction. A layer of protective denial shelters us from absorbing the news too quickly. We feel numb. Then, as our bodies adapt to the increased stress, we start to question. We want to know more.

This chapter answers questions about the testing process for hepatitis B from the time you are diagnosed through the years of ongoing care. It covers the following topics:

- Hepatitis B Virus Tests
    Proteins, Antigens, and Antibodies
    Surface Antigen (HBsAg)
    Core Antigen (HBcAg)
    e Antigen (HBeAg)
    X Protein
    DNA Polymerase
    Surface Antibody (HBsAb)
    Core Antibody (HBcAb)
    e Antibody (HBeAb)
    Hepatitis B DNA (HBV DNA)
    Case Study
    Precore Mutants
- Liver Imaging Tests
    Ultrasonography (US, Ultrasound)
    Computed Tomography (CT Scan)
    Magnetic Resonance Imaging (MRI)
- Liver Biopsy
    Biopsy Procedure
    Interpreting Biopsy Results
- Liver Blood Tests
    Liver Enzymes
    Bilirubin
    Albumin
    Clotting Factors
    Alpha-fetoprotein
    Complete Blood Count
- Patterns of Hepatitis B Tests in Patients
    Acute Hepatitis B
    Chronic Hepatitis B
    Chronic Carrier of Hepatitis B Virus
    Testing, Testing

Hepatitis B Virus Tests

When I was diagnosed in 1995, I didn't know any hepatitis B language. I couldn't figure out what the tests meant. I wrote to some organizations, but they were no help. They sent me simple little pamphlets that didn't explain enough.

Finally, I talked to medical professionals who gave me more advanced reading material. But to tell you the truth, for the first three months I lived on soda and crackers—and I was too ill to care.

Judy

Hepatitis B is a complex infection. In order to understand what your test results mean, it helps to know some facts about the virus (see Figure 2A). Before reading on, I recommend that you review the sections "What Is a Virus?" and "What Is the Hepatitis B Virus?" in Chapter 1.

Hepatitis B tests fall into three main groups. (1) Blood tests measure viral proteins, viral DNA, antibodies, and define the state of the virus in your body. These tests tell the doctor whether you have active infection or have cleared infection and are immune. (2) Liver imaging defines the size and shape of the liver and detects liver masses, such as liver cancer. (3) Other blood tests define the degree of liver injury or damage and also measure specific liver functions.

FIGURE 2A. THE HEPATITIS B VIRUS

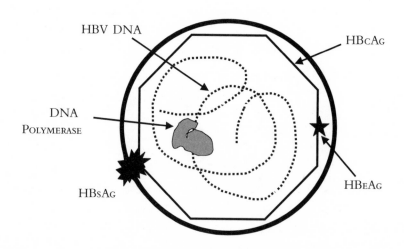

TABLE 1: TEST RESULTS FOR DIFFERENT TYPES OF
HEPATITIS B INFECTION

Test	Acute Hepatitis	Past Infection (Immunity)	Post-Vaccination	Chronic Hepatitis	Pre-Core Chronic Hepatitis	Healthy Carrier
HBsAg	+	-	-	+	+	+
HBsAb	-	+	+	-	-	-
HBcAb	+	+	-	+	+	+
HBcAb-IgM	+	-	-	-	-	-
eAg	+	-	-	+	-	-
eAb	-	+	-	-	+	+
HBV DNA	+	-	-	+/-	+/-	-
ALT	Elevated	Normal	Normal	Elevated	Elevated	Normal

Shetty, K. and Younossi, Z.M. Diagnositic Tests for Viral Hepatitis B and C. *Practical Gastroenterology* 1998; 22 (5):39-47.

Proteins, Antigens, and Antibodies. Doctors order many tests for patients with hepatitis B that measure antigens and antibodies (see Table 1). Although the terms seem complicated, a few basic definitions can help you understand your test results.

The genes of the hepatitis B virus produce five proteins: surface, core, e, X, and DNA polymerase. Three of these viral proteins or peptides (surface, core, and e) are called target antigens, because your body recognizes and targets them as foreign substances. Your immune system, which is like an army, sends protein "soldiers" (antibodies) into your bloodstream to fight these target antigens. The antibodies shape themselves to match the target antigens on the surface of the virus and in the liver. When the antibodies attach themselves to the hepatitis B virus, your body's white blood cells move in to destroy the invaders.

Surface Antigen (HBsAg). If you test positive for surface antigen (abbreviated as HBsAg in laboratory reports), it means that your liver is infected with hepatitis B and is producing this protein. In most cases, the surface antigen in your blood is a marker for the complete virus particle; both the e antigen and hepatitis B DNA are also positive, and your blood is highly infectious.

In some cases, however, surface antigen is positive but e antigen and hepatitis B DNA are negative. This means that the virus is no longer replicating (reproducing), but it still infects the liver and produces these proteins. Blood is less infectious when e antigen and DNA are negative, but the virus is still present.

If you test positive for surface antigen, you are infectious and your blood cannot be used for donation. Your body's immune system targets surface antigen, and that interaction produces surface antibody (described on p. 23).

> *At first, I found antibody and antigen test results very confusing. I finally thought of a simple way to figure it out. Here it is:*
>
> *Antigens are bad. Antibodies are good. The best possible scenario is to have two positive antibodies and two negative antigens.*
>
> *Dana*

Core Antigen (HBcAg). Core antigen, an integral component of the virus particle, typically is not measured in clinical practice. Core protein forms the coat that covers the hepatitis B DNA, as it becomes a complete virus. When the virus replicates within your liver cells, the core protein is produced. Your body's immune response to this infection produces core antibodies to the core antigen. In clinical practice, we measure core antibodies (described on p. 23).

e Antigen (HBeAg). Core protein is initially made with an extra peptide that is later split to yield the final core molecule. The cleaved peptide is called e antigen. Core and e antigens are produced only during viral replication. Therefore, we measure e antigen as a marker that indicates active, ongoing viral replication. If you test positive for e antigen, you are infected with hepatitis B, and the virus is actively reproducing.

X Protein. The exact role of X protein is unclear, but it may assist in the integration of hepatitis B DNA into the body's cellular DNA. Scientists think this step may be a factor in the development of hepatocellular carcinoma (liver cancer). We do not measure X protein in clinical practice.

DNA Polymerase. DNA polymerase is an enzyme that promotes the production of hepatitis B DNA and is essential for viral replication. It is a component of the viral particle and is also produced during active infection. Prior to assays for hepatitis B DNA, its measurement was used as a surrogate marker for DNA replication and viral replication. Tests of DNA polymerase are no longer used in clinical practice.

Surface Antibody (HBsAb). Your body's immune response to surface antigen produces surface antibody. It is a marker of viral eradication and lifelong immunity.

Patients can have surface antibody either from prior exposure to and clearance of hepatitis B infection or from prior vaccination with hepatitis B vaccine. Patients who were previously exposed to hepatitis B infection and who develop surface antibody have cleared the infection and test negative for surface antigen, e antigen, and hepatitis B DNA. These patients will also test positive for antibodies to core and e antigens.

Because surface antibody indicates immunity, researchers aimed their efforts to produce a hepatitis B vaccine at the surface antigen. Hepatitis B vaccines are either extracts or synthetic derivatives of surface antigen. For this reason, vaccinated patients test positive for surface antibody. But, in contrast to natural infection, they do not make antibodies against core and e antigens.

Rarely, a patient with chronic hepatitis B will have an immune response that produces low levels of surface antibody. These patients will test positive for both surface antigen and surface antibody.

Core Antibody (HBcAb). Core antibodies, produced in response to hepatitis B infection, are not protective and do not indicate immunity. These antibodies simply mark past or current infection.

We measure two classes of core antibodies: IgG and IgM. Patients who resolve the infection produce IgG antibodies but also have surface antibody, the true marker for immunity. In contrast, patients with chronic hepatitis B who have ongoing infection and lack surface antibody also produce IgG core antibodies. IgM antibodies are found primarily during initial infection with the virus and are a very important diagnostic test for acute hepatitis B.

e Antibody (HBeAb). The body produces the e antibody in one of two ways: (1) temporarily, during an acute infection or (2) in a sustained way during or after a flare. A flare occurs when patients with chronic hepatitis B have an immune response to a burst in viral replication. During a flare, the patient experiences a rise in ALT, positive e antigen, and positive hepatitis B DNA.

The immune response may spontaneously generate the e antibody and lead to a resolution in hepatic inflammation. Spontaneous seroconversion (a spontaneous change in blood serum from e antigen to e antibody) rarely, if ever, leads to clearing the virus. Patients who undergo this e antigen to e antibody conversion (sometimes referred to as "flip-flop") may also revert back to positive e antigen. In contrast, during antiviral therapy with either interferon or lamivudine, the conversion of e antigen to e antibody is a predictor of long-term clearance of the virus (see Chapter 8).

I'm one of those crazy people whose e antigen disappears only to have it reappear again! It's been gone now for two years. And after all those years I haven't developed antibodies.

Julie

Hepatitis B DNA (HBV DNA). Hepatitis B is a DNA virus (see Chapter 1). DNA, deoxyribonucleic acid, is the backbone for the genes of the virus and directs the manufacture of the virus's proteins. The finding of hepatitis B DNA in blood indicates active viral replication. High levels correlate with high replication rates of the virus.

However, there is no direct correlation between levels of hepatitis B DNA and degree of liver injury. Some patients with very high DNA levels lack evidence of liver injury, while others with low levels may have substantial damage. Doctors use hepatitis B DNA levels to monitor response to antiviral therapy. If your hepatitis B DNA levels disappear by the time your treatment ends, we say that you have achieved remission.

Case Study. Here's an example of "test interpretation" in a patient who had acute hepatitis B, cleared the infection, and now has positive antibodies.

In 1971, I had an emergency Cesarean section. I lost the baby. The doctors gave me a blood transfusion and fibrinogen to save my life. A week or so later, I had hepatitis and was jaundiced, nauseous, and run-down. I couldn't eat.

One year ago I had blood work that turned up positive for hepatitis B. And recently, I went for an annual checkup that showed my bilirubin was elevated to 1.9 milligrams per deciliter (nearly all the bilirubin was "unconjugated"). The rest of my liver tests were normal. My doctor repeated the hepatitis B tests: surface antigen negative, surface antibody positive, core antibody positive.

What do the tests mean? Do I have hepatitis B? Is my liver damaged?

Annie

Annie clearly had a bout of acute hepatitis in 1971. However, she cleared the infection and developed antibodies (surface and core). Annie no longer is infected or infectious, and she is immune to hepatitis B.

Her liver enzymes are normal so she lacks evidence of liver injury, but her bilirubin is elevated. Bilirubin is a pigment in the blood, created from the breakdown of red blood cells and cleared from the blood by the liver (see p. 32). Clearance of bilirubin is dependent upon specific liver functions, one of which conjugates (binds) the bilirubin to another molecule so it can be excreted from the body.

The fact that most of Annie's bilirubin is unconjugated means that she has an abnormality in the liver's ability to conjugate bilirubin, a condition called Gilbert's syndrome. Gilbert's syndrome is a genetically-acquired trait, occurs in 1 to 3 percent of the population, and is not associated with liver damage.

Precore Mutants. Sometimes the hepatitis B virus is actively replicating, but e antigen is negative—a condition called precore mutation (see Chapter 8). Patients with this mutation (spontaneous change) in the hepatitis B virus are positive for surface antigen, produce core antibody, have positive hepatitis B DNA, but lack e antigen. The mutation produces a defective e antigen that no longer reacts to clinical assays.

Liver Imaging Tests

Don't be alarmed if your doctor orders a radiologic imaging test, such as an ultrasound or a computed tomography (CT) scan. The tests are non-invasive and give information about your liver.

Ultrasonography (US, Ultrasound). Ultrasonography is a safe and painless way to investigate the size, structure, and the vascular (blood) supply of the liver. It's the preferred radiologic technique for an initial assessment for liver tumors.

Ultrasonic waves penetrate the body tissues, and a recording device picks up reflected sound waves that yield an image of the liver. You can compare it to exploring for oil by using seismographic recordings of the earth's formations.

Here's what ultrasound helps find out: liver size and texture and the size of bile ducts and blood vessels. Doppler probes added to ultrasound can detect direction and rates of blood flow in vessels going to and from the liver. Your physician may order ultrasound to pinpoint the liver's location just before a biopsy.

Computed Tomography (CT Scan). Unlike ultrasound, computed tomography (CT scan) uses a highly sophisticated X-ray machine to scan the internal organs with minimal radiation. CT scans are used to confirm the findings of ultrasound and to get a clearer view because, unlike ultrasound, CT scans aren't blocked by air in the bowel. The scans are also more standardized and much less dependent on the expertise of the technician performing the test. CT scans define the size and texture of the liver and can detect an early liver tumor (see Figure 2B).

Magnetic Resonance Imaging (MRI). Unlike ultrasound and CT scans, MRI measures special signals from the body's water molecules.

FIGURE 2B. CT SCANS OF NORMAL LIVER, CIRRHOTIC LIVER, AND
LIVER TUMOR (HEPATOMA)

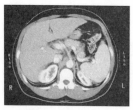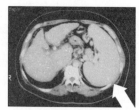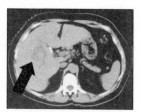

| NONCIRRHOTIC | CIRRHOTIC | LIVER CANCER (HEPATOMA) |

LEGEND 2B: CT scans are specialized radiologic tests that allow one to peer inside the abdomen. The image on the left demonstrates a normal liver and spleen. The middle panel depicts a liver with a knobby irregular surface and an enlarged spleen (⇨) in a cirrhotic patient. The image to the right shows a liver cancer (hepatoma) in the middle of the liver(➡). The patient with the cancer was treated by chemoembolization of the tumor and liver transplantation and is currently alive without evidence of tumor.

Images are created from these signals. Magnetic resonance imaging is used mainly to diagnose liver cancers.

Liver Biopsy

Just the word "biopsy" strikes fear into people's hearts, but it's an essential part of your evaluation and may determine type of treatment. Only a biopsy can give your doctor a true idea of the condition of your liver. You need a biopsy for two reasons:

1. It confirms the diagnosis and rules out other disorders, such as granulomatous liver disease, infections, or biliary tract disorders. Liver biopsy along with ultrasound or a CT scan can be used to pinpoint the site of a lesion and rule out liver cancers.
2. It establishes the stage and degree of activity of hepatitis B. Typically, chronic viral hepatitis passes in sequence from a mild inflammatory stage to fibrosis and, later, cirrhosis. Biopsies may be done over many years to record the progression. Once cirrhosis has developed, there is little reason to continue the biopsies.

Biopsy Procedure. Years ago, liver biopsies often required a short hospital stay. Today it's an outpatient procedure that literally takes seconds. In fact, you'll spend most of your time getting ready for the biopsy and being monitored after the biopsy has been done. The whole procedure requires approximately four hours. However, it is invasive, and you will be asked to sign an informed consent form. It's a good idea to select a doctor who frequently performs this procedure and is very familiar with it. Biopsies may be performed every three to five years.

Here's one patient's experience with liver biopsy:

> I was nervous about having a biopsy because of what that word means to most people, but it turned out to be a simple procedure. I knew I had to remain very still when they did it so I requested something to help me relax. It took longer for the drug to take effect than for the biopsy itself. The doctor poked a needle through my side and boom—it was over. In and out. Thirty seconds. A vaccination is more painful.
>
> The longest part of the whole thing was the nurses checking on my paperwork, and explaining what they were going to do. The doctor was in and out of there in about five minutes. I spent more time with the nurses than with the doctor. They told me it was a good idea to rest after-

wards, because essentially they were puncturing an organ. I went home and spent a quiet day.

Tom

As you can see from Tom's story, most patients' fears come from not knowing what to expect. Here's how the procedure goes:

Your physician examines you carefully to decide exactly where to place the biopsy needle and cleanses the skin with iodine or an antiseptic solution. Then you'll get a local anesthetic, as you do at the dentist's, at the spot where the biopsy needle will be placed. Some doctors also prescribe intravenous benzodiazepine with a narcotic to lessen the anxiety and discomfort.

You'll feel strong pressure when the needle is inserted, but the whole procedure takes only a few seconds for a small core of tissue to be obtained. Then you'll be rolled onto your right side to help control any bleeding from the surface of the liver. You'll stay in the procedure area for two to four hours for observation. If you're stable, with no symptoms, you'll be discharged.

After performing biopsies on thousands of patients, I've seen very few complications. Reported rates vary from 1 percent to 0.1 percent. If the most common complication occurs, bleeding from the surface of the liver, the patient may require transfusions or even an operation. In rare cases, the biopsy needle may pierce another organ, such as the bowel, gallbladder, kidney, or lung. Serious complications are very rare, occurring in less than one in 1,000 cases.

Interpreting Biopsy Results. Your doctor will tell you the results of your biopsy in terms of histologic stages. Histology means the examination of tissue under the microscope. There are four histologic stages in liver injury due to hepatitis B:

- **Stage I** is characterized by inflammation without the development of any scar tissue.
- **Stage II** features include inflammation with early scarring (fibrosis) in one zone (portal) of the liver.
- **Stage III** shows bridging of the fibrosis between adjacent portal tracts.
- **Stage IV** is cirrhosis (advanced scarring with loss of normal liver architecture).

FIGURE 2C. HISTOLOGIC STAGES OF HEPATITIS B

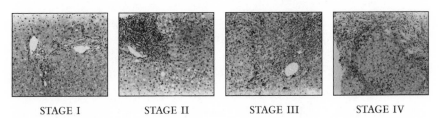

| STAGE I | STAGE II | STAGE III | STAGE IV |

LEGEND 2C: This figure demonstrates the progressive microscopic changes that may occur in livers infected with viral hepatitis. Stage I shows only mild inflammation in the portal tract; stage II exhibits more inflammation with spread of fibrosis (scar tissue) into adjacent liver cells; stage III implies that fibrosis has spread between portal tracts; stage IV is cirrhosis with formation of nodules.

Histologic stages don't correspond very well to the duration of infection. For example, a patient with slowly progressive disease may maintain an early histologic stage for many years or even decades. Another patient may progress to cirrhosis in less than a decade. The stages of liver damage are distinctive under the microscope (see Figure 2C).

Physicians use certain specific terms when interpreting liver biopsies from patients with hepatitis B. Here's a quick translation:

Stage of Disease	Terminology
Early stage, mild activity (I)	Chronic Persistent Hepatitis B or Mild Chronic Active Hepatitis B
Intermediate stage (II or III)	Chronic Active Hepatitis B with Fibrosis
Advanced stage (IV)	Cirrhosis

Liver Blood Tests

Life with hepatitis B means lots of blood tests to monitor your condition. Have you ever wondered what the numbers really mean? Read the next few pages to understand these tests and to review the warning signals when the tests are abnormal:

1. enzymes
2. bilirubin
3. albumin

4. clotting factors
5. complete blood count

Doctors test blood so frequently in viral hepatitis patients because blood tests warn of changes. The most informative tests "dip" into this bloodstream to measure liver injury (enzymes) or assess liver function (bilirubin, albumin, clotting factors, complete blood count). At first, you may feel intimidated by medical terminology, acronyms, and numbers, but learning about these basic tests will help you understand your doctor's interpretation of results (see Table 2).

TABLE 2. NORMAL AND ABNORMAL VALUES FOR LABORATORY TESTS

Test	Normal Range	Abnormal Range	
		Mild to Moderate	Severe
Liver Enzymes			
AST	< 40 IU/L	40–200	> 200
ALT	< 40 IU/L	40–200	> 200
GGT	< 60 IU/L	60–200	> 200
Alkaline Phosphatase	<112 IU/L	112–300	> 300
Liver Function Tests			
Bilirubin	< 1.2 mg/dl	1.2–2.5	> 2.5
Albumin	3.5–4.5 g/dl	3.0–3.5	< 3.0
Prothrombin Time	< 14 seconds	14–17	> 17
Blood Count			
WBC	> 6000	3000–6000	< 3000
HCT	> 40	35–40	< 35
Platelets	> 150,000	100,000–150,000	< 100,000

KEY:
IU = International Units
l = liter
dl = deciliter
mg = milligrams
AST (SGOT) = aspartate aminotransferase
ALT (SGPT) = alanine aminotransferase
GGT = gamma-glutamyl transferase
WBC = white blood count
HCT = hematocrit (percentage of blood occupied by red blood cells)

The blood test results and numbers can get pretty complicated. I used to keep track of only ALT and AST results and dates. Now I know that all the liver function tests are important and give information about how my liver is handling the infection.

I ask for copies of all my tests now, and I keep them on file at home. It helps me feel more in control, as if I'm somehow staying on top of things.

When you're sick, you feel helpless. Then you get depressed. You have to switch to taking a more active role in your care.

Sally

Liver Enzymes. A liver cell produces proteins, called enzymes, that live within the cell or its membranes. In a way, you can think of your liver as a powerful chemical factory; it changes raw materials into the substances your body needs. Enzymes are catalysts that help a liver cell do its job of creating the specific chemical changes that give your body fuel to live. Here are the names of the enzymes you need to remember:

- ALT (SGPT)—alanine aminotransferase
- AST (SGOT)—aspartate aminotransferase
- GGT—gamma-glutamyl transferase
- alkaline phosphatase

By measuring the level of these enzymes in your blood, doctors can monitor ongoing liver injury. Why? Under normal conditions, the level of these enzymes in your bloodstream is relatively low. But when liver cells are injured, destroyed, or die, the cell becomes leaky, and the enzymes escape into the blood that's circulating through the liver. When the cell is injured, liver enzyme levels in the blood rise.

Massive liver injury is associated with marked increases in ALT; mild injury may be associated with mild—or even no—increase in ALT. The correlation is strongest at earlier stages of hepatitis B, before the development of cirrhosis. After cirrhosis occurs, however, ALT levels may not be high and therefore no longer serve as a good indicator of further liver damage.

What do the numbers mean? Table 2 shows normal and abnormal test values. Blood test patterns relate somewhat to the type of liver injury. Typical hepatitis B patients show increases in ALT and AST but little or no increase in GGT and alkaline phosphatase. Those with cirrhosis or who have an underlying disorder of the biliary tract (the ducts that drain bile from the liver into the intestine) may have modest elevations in GGT and alkaline phosphatase. In some unusual cases of hepatitis B, I have even seen a predominant elevation in GGT.

Patients tend to focus on their ALT and AST counts, but other tests are more important in measuring the health of your liver.

Bilirubin. When red blood cells complete their life cycle and break down naturally in your body, they produce a yellow pigment that's passed to the liver and excreted into bile. Bile helps your body digest food, but the pigment, which has no digestive function, is called bilirubin. Blood levels of bilirubin tend to fluctuate in patients with hepatitis, although a prolonged persistent elevation in bilirubin usually means severe liver dysfunction and possibly cirrhosis.

Here's why. Most of the time, the body produces as many red blood cells as it breaks down, so you produce a constant amount of bilirubin. However, if your blood cells break down more rapidly (hemolysis) or your liver function becomes impaired, the bilirubin levels in your blood rise.

Your liver has to go to work to take up the excess bilirubin into the liver cell, metabolize it to make it more water-soluble for excretion into bile, and send it through special passages and ducts into the intestine. Microbes in the gut continue to metabolize the bilirubin until you expel it. (Stercobilin, a brown pigment derived from bilirubin, creates the dark brown color of feces.)

When the liver fails to eliminate bilirubin from the blood, the skin and whites of the eyes turn yellow (jaundice), urine darkens, and the color of the bowel movement lightens. In case you've wondered, now you know why your doctor asks you probing questions about the color of your feces.

Albumin. Albumin is another protein synthesized (manufactured) by the liver. Liver cells secrete albumin to maintain the volume of blood in arteries and veins. When albumin levels drop to extremely low levels, fluid may leak out of the blood vessels into the surrounding tissues. This causes swelling, known as edema. Normal albumin levels range between 3.5 to 4.5 grams/deciliter. Usually, edema occurs when levels drop below 2.5 grams/deciliter.

Unlike liver enzyme increases, which occur within hours to days of the liver injury, albumin levels don't fall unless there has been chronic progressive liver injury for at least one month or more. This is because albumin has a long residence time in the plasma; its half life is approximately 20 days. A decrease in serum albumin, therefore, reflects a slowly progressive, ongoing reduction in the liver's ability to synthesize this protein.

Be aware that there are non-liver reasons for albumin to decrease and your physician will take these into account when interpreting test results. Nonetheless, a significant sustained decrease in serum albumin may mean poor liver function and cirrhosis of the liver. Patients with very low albumin counts may need to be considered for liver transplantation.

Clotting Factors. Remember our comparison of the liver to a chemical factory? The liver also synthesizes many proteins that maintain normal blood clotting. Prothrombin time (PT) is the name of the most common test that measures a combination of blood clotting factors. If your prothrombin time increases, it means your liver isn't creating enough factors, so it takes your blood longer to clot.

Unlike albumin, clotting factors can decrease rapidly—within days, or even hours, of a severe liver injury. In severe cases, clotting disturbances may signal the need for an early transplant. In patients with chronic hepatitis and chronic liver disease, a prolonged prothrombin time can be a warning that the liver is having trouble with its synthetic functions.

> I had a nosebleed that lasted, off and on, for two weeks. Three times I went to the emergency room bleeding buckets. Finally, they fixed it.
> Then the doctors put me on lamivudine. I've been on it ever since, and my prothrombin time improved—15 seconds. My internal coagulation time, the APPT score, went from 52 to 40. No more nosebleeds.
>
> *Sam*

Typically, doctors will administer Vitamin K, a vitamin essential for normal clotting factors, to determine whether the clotting disorder is reversible. Patients who have persistent, prolonged elevations in prothrombin time that don't respond to Vitamin K may need to be considered for liver transplantation.

Alpha-Fetoprotein. This is a protein that regenerative cells or cancer cells secrete into blood. Increased blood levels of alpha-fetoprotein may indicate the development of liver cancer (see Chapter 10).

Complete Blood Count. The complete blood count test can be a detection system for liver scarring. Here's how. Blood from your spleen flows through your liver via the portal vein. When the liver becomes scarred, it creates resistance to this blood flow (called portal hypertension), and the blood may back up into the spleen. When this happens, the spleen enlarges and traps blood elements, removing them from circulation and lowering blood counts.

Although all components of the blood count may decrease, those most sensitive to this condition are the white blood cell and platelet counts. Patients with portal hypertension from cirrhosis of the liver often have low counts. Similarly, patients may have an enlarged spleen, resulting from severe cirrhotic disease, and may need to be considered for liver transplantation.

Patterns of Hepatitis B Tests in Patients

Acute Hepatitis B. Acute hepatitis occurs 30 to 90 days after infection with the hepatitis B virus. Most patients don't have jaundice and other symptoms during this incubation period. Their liver tests are normal. Some patients, however, experience fever, joint pain, and a hives-like skin rash. These symptoms and signs are called the prodrome prior to the development of clinical liver injury—hepatitis.

The onset of hepatitis is associated with flu-like symptoms, low-grade fever, abnormal liver tests, and jaundice. Acutely ill patients test positive for surface antigen and IgM core antibody (Table 1). In clinical practice, doctors typically don't measure other markers of hepatitis B, such as e antigen and antibody, surface antibody, and hepatitis B DNA, nor do we find imaging studies of the liver useful unless we suspect underlying chronic disease. Similarly, doctors don't usually do a liver biopsy unless we're concerned about underlying or pre-existing chronic liver disease.

Ninety to 95 percent of these patients will clear the infection. Symptoms resolve, ALT and bilirubin normalize, surface antigen disappears, and surface antibody develops (see Figure 2D). Surface antibody persists for life and is a marker of immunity. Re-exposure to hepatitis B does not cause infection or disease.

Chronic Hepatitis B. Five to 10 percent of adult patients with acute hepatitis B fail to clear infection and develop chronic infection. Most of these patients experience ongoing evidence of liver injury with abnor-

FIGURE 2D: COURSE OF ACUTE HEPATITIS B WITH RESOLUTION
OF INFECTION

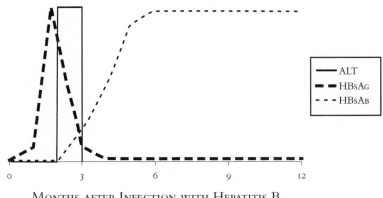

MONTHS AFTER INFECTION WITH HEPATITIS B

LEGEND 2D: This figure shows the course of acute resolving hepatitis B, assuming infection with virus at month 0. In this case, a two-month incubation period precedes development of hepatitis. Abnormal ALT signals onset and resolution of hepatitis (solid line). Surface antigen (HBsAg) is positive prior to onset of liver injury and rise in ALT and begins to clear during the hepatitic phase. In most cases of acute resolving hepatitis B, the surface antigen is negative when the ALT has normalized. Surface antibody begins to rise with clearance of surface antigen and remains positive for life.

mal liver enzymes and have persistent viral infection with positive surface antigen, e antigen, and hepatitis B DNA (see Table 1 and Figure 2E).

> My blood counts had been fluctuating drastically for two to three years. I went to see the doctor for back pain. He took a blood test, and it came back positive for hepatitis B. I wasn't surprised—not really. My mother and my two aunts died from hepatitis B. I thought gosh, that virus has got to be in there somewhere.

> Max

Flares in disease activity, characterized by abrupt elevations in ALT, are often accompanied by flu-like symptoms and even jaundice. For this

FIGURE 2E: COURSE OF CHRONIC HEPATITIS B DEVELOPING AFTER ACUTE INFECTION

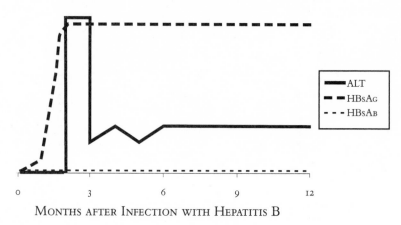

MONTHS AFTER INFECTION WITH HEPATITIS B

LEGEND 2E: This figure shows the course of chronic hepatitis B, assuming infection with virus at month 0. Surface antigen (HBsAg) persists and surface antibody (HBsAb) fails to develop. ALT remains elevated but typically at lower levels than observed during acute hepatitis. These patients also have positive e antigen, hepatitis B DNA, and core antibody (not shown).

reason, doctors may mistakenly diagnose a case of chronic hepatitis B as acute hepatitis B. Patients with chronic hepatitis B, however, fail to develop surface antibody.

Imaging studies and liver biopsy evaluate the stage of disease and detect cirrhosis and liver cancer. The risk of liver cancer is greatest in those with cirrhosis.

Chronic Carrier of Hepatitis B Virus. The likelihood of developing the carrier state is related to age at the time of infection. In the absence of preventive therapy, the transmission of hepatitis B from mother to infant at the time of delivery leads to chronic infection in 75 to 85 percent of cases. Most of these babies and children lack evidence for liver injury, have normal ALT levels, and are classified as carriers.

These patients are still at risk for liver cancer if they carry the infection for 20 to 30 years. We recommend screening for liver cancer using alpha-fetoprotein and ultrasonography for patients who have carried hepatitis B for 20 or more years.

The risk of developing chronic hepatitis B after an initial acute attack of HBV diminishes with age at the time of exposure: 85 percent for

FIGURE 2F: COURSE OF CHRONIC CARRIER DEVELOPING AFTER ACUTE INFECTION

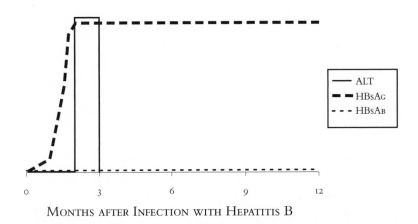

——— ALT
▬ ▬ HBsAg
- - - HBsAb

MONTHS AFTER INFECTION WITH HEPATITIS B

LEGEND 2F: This figure shows the course of the chronic carrier developing after acute infection. These patients are characterized by persistently positive surface antigen (HBsAg) and lack surface antibody (HBsAb). In contrast to patients with chronic hepatitis, ALT is normal, indicating lack of liver injury.

newborns, 50 percent for infants, 25 percent for children up to age 13, and 5 to 10 percent for adolescents and adults. Carriers show a consistent test pattern: positive surface antigen with or without markers of viral replication, normal ALT, normal liver function, and normal liver biopsy (see Table 1 and Figure 2F).

Testing, Testing. In the past few years, I've seen the advancement of specific new tests that help monitor your health. But all too often I find that patients feel shut out by the complicated language of test results. Don't worry if you didn't absorb every detail. Use these pages as a reference guide.

Ask for copies of your tests. When you have questions, look up the answers in these pages. Often, your physician can calm your fears if you voice them. Talk with your doctor.

Knowledge is power.

Francis Bacon

3

WHY ME?
WHAT ABOUT THEM?

How You Got Infected and How to Avoid Infecting Others

I was in a relationship for eleven years. My girlfriend's former hus-band used I.V. drugs and contracted hepatitis B somewhere down the line. He told my girlfriend she should get tested, and she found out she had it, too.

I went through blaming myself, my partner. I was angry. It's a nat-ural process, and you have to get through it. You have to get through the blame. I don't really know who gave it to whom. I had other part-ners before Carol. Did I get it from her or give it to her?

Finally, I resolved that it was a life lesson, and apparently I'm not getting off that easy. I've got some rough lessons to learn.

I still have some temper tantrums, but it's getting better.

Robert

WHEN YOU'RE DEALING with a serious illness, it's the most human thing in the world to ask, "Why me? What did I do to get hepatitis B?"

The answer is both simple and complex. You acquired hepatitis B when you came into direct contact with blood or body fluids infected with the virus, and the virus gained entry into your bloodstream.

Only one-third of adults (10 percent of young children) have symptoms of hepatitis B when they are first infected. If you can't recall an initial illness, your liver disease may go undetected for 20 to 40 years and you may have no idea how you contracted the virus.

On the other hand, you may recall risky behaviors that give you some possible clues. In the United States the three major risk factors for hepatitis B are intravenous (I.V.) drug use, male homosexual activity, and emigration from a region of the world with a high prevalence of hepatitis B.

How did you get hepatitis B? And how can you avoid giving the virus to others? We'll discuss ways to protect your family and friends. In addition, we'll provide up-to-date summaries of documented ways that hepatitis B is transmitted, including:

- Overview: How Infectious Is Hepatitis B?
- Intravenous Drug Abuse
- Sexual Transmission
- Birth and Delivery
- Immigrants and Travelers from Countries with High Rates of HBV
- Transfusion of Blood or Blood Products
    Surgery or Medical Treatment
    Hemophilia
- Needle-Stick Accidents
- Tattooing and Body Piercing
- Household Contact/Casual Contact
- Institutional Contact
- Organ Transplantation
- How Can I Avoid Infecting Others?

Overview: How Infectious Is Hepatitis B?

Hepatitis B-infected blood is 50 to 100 times more infectious than HIV-infected blood. This means that if you compare one drop of blood, the drop of blood with hepatitis B virus would have 50 to 100 times more virus particles in it. The virus also lives for several days on surfaces it touches. Obviously, hepatitis B has a lot of "power" to infect.

If you're infected, it's hard not to feel dirty or contaminated. You cannot control how you got the virus in the past, but you *can* help stop the spread of this disease today. You are an army of one, and you can protect others by taking the precautions described in this chapter. Urge your family and friends to get vaccinated. Close contacts may need an injection of Hepatitis B Immune Globulin (HBIG) plus vaccine. Use universal precautions. Cover hands with gloves when cleaning infected blood spills or dirty diapers. Inform sexual partners of effective vaccines. Practice safe sex by using latex condoms, and avoid the risky behaviors described in this chapter.

The hepatitis B virus exists in the blood and body fluids of an infected person. For you to infect others, your blood, saliva, semen, or vaginal secretions have to get into their bloodstreams. How does this occur?

Intravenous Drug Abuse

What's the most direct way to get hepatitis B? Inoculate the virus from infected blood into your own bloodstream. That's why one of the most common risk factors is a history of using intravenous illicit drugs. Many drug addicts share needles. They spread hepatitis among themselves and maintain a pool of infected people. Studies suggest that more than 75 percent of current or past heavy users of intravenous drugs have been exposed to hepatitis B.

Although some patients recollect an episode of jaundice, and others report significant past drug use, many don't have a clue how they got the virus. I ask them if they've experimented with intravenous drugs. They're shocked. "Can that do it?" they'll say. "It was only once or twice."

In many cases we can't identify a risk factor for hepatitis B. Some doctors think that most of these cases are due to prior use of intravenous drugs. People who are otherwise healthy, employed, and raising their families are stunned to hear they have hepatitis B. They can't believe the diagnosis relates to a past, seemingly insignificant experiment so long ago.

"I don't know how I could get hepatitis B from sharing needles. I was always so careful about cleaning them," patients often say. But to understand how contamination occurs, you have to appreciate how concentrated the virus is in the blood of infected patients.

The average patient with chronic hepatitis B has a blood concentration of the virus of one billion particles per milliliter of whole blood. That's equivalent to 1,000,000 particles of virus in the amount of blood that would sit on the head of a small stickpin. With this concentration it's easy to see that wiping or rinsing a needle with water or salt solutions won't remove all the virus particles. Indeed, a large amount of virus may remain on the needle.

A concentrated solution of hydrogen peroxide will kill or inactivate the virus, and cleaning needles with this solution may reduce the risk of transmission. It won't protect you, however, if cleaning is superficial, such as a quick rinse, or if the internal chamber of the needle is not irrigated and the syringe and all its external and internal parts are not cleansed. Some people rely on others to clean a syringe and don't realize that it's not done thoroughly.

We Americans face a tremendous public health problem from illegal drug use. According to the 1999 National Household Survey on Drug Abuse, 6.4 million Americans age 12 and older reported using illicit drugs (other than or with marijuana and hashish) during the month prior to the interview. An estimated 1.5 million currently used cocaine, and an estimated 200,000 currently used heroin.

On a personal level, the risk factor rises each time you use drugs. If you shoot up once, you may or may not get hepatitis B. But if you shoot up many times, you can almost count on it. The best way to avoid the risk is to avoid illicit intravenous drugs and to teach the next generation to avoid this dangerous behavior.

Although not proven, snorting cocaine could potentially transmit hepatitis B. Intranasal use of cocaine causes constriction of the blood vessels in the mucous membrane of the nose, leading to disruption of the lining and ulceration. A well-known consequence of chronic cocaine use is necrosis of the nasal septum, leaving a hole in the cartilage that separates the two nostrils. Sharing straws during cocaine use, therefore, is a possible (but not proven) route of blood-to-blood transmission of hepatitis B. Researchers have not investigated cocaine use and hepatitis B, although a recent epidemiological study[1] for risk factors for hepatitis C highly correlated hepatitis C with patients who were regular users of cocaine.

Sexual Transmission

Hepatitis B pretty much kills sex—unless you've got a vaccinated partner. The virus shows up in all body fluids so even French kissing is out. How do you know if your partner has a cut in her mouth so that your saliva can infect her? If you really want to be safe, you need an inoculated partner.

I care about anybody I'm involved with and their well-being. If you care, you protect the other person. That's just human decency.

Alan

This is one of the most sensitive and troubling topics for patients. Condoms reduce the risk of hepatitis B infection, but that is not enough. Sexual hepatitis B partners can be completely protected by the use of immune globulin (HBIG) and vaccination.

Singles have troubling issues. How do you start an intimate relationship without being honest about hepatitis B? And how will the other person react? Current treatments can completely protect a sexual partner. It's your responsibility to inform your partner of your condition and the availability of preventive measures.

There are two effective treatments. HBIG contains antibody that binds hepatitis B and *immediately* inactivates it. Persons who receive HBIG are immediately protected from infection for approximately 30 days. The other treatment, hepatitis B vaccine, induces your immune system to produce antibodies, but this reaction takes time. Typically, patients require three doses of vaccine given over a six-month period to be fully protected. Doctors can test for antibody protection at any time during or after this vaccination schedule to determine if you've developed a protective antibody response.

The main goal of these treatments is to develop and maintain surface antibody, which means you are immune to hepatitis B. Confirm that you have produced antibodies by testing your blood for surface antibody after completing the vaccination schedule (see Chapter 8).

Who is most at risk sexually and why? High risk sexual behaviors include unprotected sex, multiple sexual partners, and homosexual activity. Studies suggest that sexual transmission of hepatitis B is more frequent in homosexual males or highly promiscuous heterosexuals. Some sexual practices are more traumatic to body tissues. For example, anal intercourse may disrupt the lining of the rectum and allow blood and body fluids containing hepatitis B to enter the blood of a sexual partner.

Birth and Delivery

If you have hepatitis B and you're pregnant or planning a family, of course you're concerned about giving birth to a healthy baby. The period of risk occurs at delivery when the mother's and baby's blood may become intermixed.

Once again, transmission from mother to baby can be prevented in more than 95 percent of cases by administering Hepatitis B Immune Globulin and vaccination to the infant at the time of delivery.

Mothers with hepatitis B often ask whether they can transmit the virus to their baby through breastfeeding. Existing information suggests that hepatitis B is rarely—if ever—transmitted to an infant through breast milk. Even though hepatitis B may be detected in breast milk, it's likely that the baby's digestive juices and enzymes would destroy the virus. The current recommendation by the American Academy of Pediatrics is that breastfeeding of a vaccinated infant poses no additional risk (see Chapter 12).

Immigrants and Travelers from Countries with High Rates of Hepatitis B

I was number eight in the family—the baby. When I was 22, I came to the United States—a little shy country boy. I was proud of my work. I used to lift 100-pound slabs of marble, and I was the foreman of 10-15 guys.

I have a strong feeling that what killed my liver was that I worked with epoxy fumes and acids. There was no protection then. Also, we used to make our own wine in Italy, and it was a tradition to drink a glass of wine with every meal.

But the doctor thinks I got it from my mother. He says hepatitis B is common in Europe, and my mother probably passed it to me. She died many years ago of liver cancer.

Rico

Hepatitis B is often imported into the United States as people immigrate from high risk areas, such as sub-Saharan Africa, most of Asia and the Pacific rim, the Amazon, southern parts of Eastern and Central Europe, portions of the Middle East, and the Indian sub-continent. Even though the U.S. has a universal vaccination program, many other parts of the world with the highest prevalence of hepatitis B don't. Therefore, immigration maintains a pool of infected individuals. Most infected immigrants acquire hepatitis B during the newborn or early childhood period rather than from risky behaviors. If you are planning to adopt children from a high risk region of the world, consider testing them for hepatitis B.

Transfusion of Blood or Blood Products

American blood banks were mandated by the FDA to routinely test for hepatitis B in 1972. As screening tests improved, the risk of contracting the virus diminished. Prior to sensitive testing, 0.3 to 1.7 percent of transfused patients developed hepatitis B. The blood supply is now much safer; current risk is extremely low. Only one in 63,000 units of blood can transmit hepatitis B. This minimum risk could be even further reduced by the use of highly sensitive polymerase chain reaction (PCR) tests.

Surgery or Medical Treatment. Prior to sensitive blood screening tests, certain medical procedures and operations were particularly associated with risk of acquiring hepatitis B due to the large number of transfusions required. These included hemodialysis, coronary artery bypass or heart surgery, lung resection, and major abdominal surgery.

> *I was born premature, a preemie with heart defects, 45 years ago. My folks had to move across from the hospital because I would turn blue from lack of oxygen and need to go to the emergency room. I was minutes from death.*
>
> *I'm not a drug user, and I'm not promiscuous so I think the platelets they gave me during heart surgery were the source of my hepatitis B.*
>
> *It's one of the cards I got dealt—the way the cookie crumbles. I have to deal with it.*
>
> *Helen*

Hemophilia. People with hemophilia lack certain clotting factors in their blood. In the past hemophiliacs were treated with plasma from a large number of donors. The plasma was combined and treated to extract those clotting factors.

Until the mid-1980s, hemophiliacs were at extreme risk for getting hepatitis B and HIV. Therefore, scientists pasteurized the clotting factor for hemophiliacs and this treatment inactivated the hepatitis B virus. Studies showed that hemophiliacs treated with the pasteurized preparation had an extremely low risk, approaching zero percent. Today, current therapy often uses synthesized or genetically engineered clotting products with a zero risk of transmitting hepatitis B.

> We knew David had hemophilia when he was six months old. He was bruising and had bleeds so the doctors gave him injections of clotting factor. When he was 16 months old, he became dehydrated and ran a high fever. We took him to the hospital. That was in 1981—before they knew there were hepatitis viruses in the clotting factor. Sure enough, he was having an acute attack of hepatitis B.
>
> Since the third grade, David has known how to inject himself in a vein with the clotting factor whenever he gets a bleed. Last year he had 87 bleeds.
>
> We never kept the hepatitis a secret because we didn't want people to whisper, whisper. We didn't want him to feel he had done something bad. We live in a small town, and everyone knows. They always ask how it's going, and they pray for us.
>
> Jackie

Needle-Stick Accidents

Health care workers face an occupational hazard: needle-stick accidents. According to the Centers for Disease Control and Prevention, 600,000 to 800,000 health workers accidentally stick themselves every year.

Because many hospitalized patients and people who frequent emergency rooms have hepatitis, medical personnel run high risks if they accidentally get stuck with an infected needle, which can easily pierce rubber gloves. In one study of an inner city emergency room at Johns Hopkins Hospital in Baltimore, MD, 24 percent of 2,523 patients over age 15 were infected with at least one of three viruses: hepatitis C (18 percent), HIV (6 percent), or hepatitis B (5 percent). Of all the patients who were bleeding and who had invasive procedures performed, 30 percent had at least one virus.

This study shows the potential exposure of medical personnel to hepatitis infection. HIV testing alone failed to identify 87 percent of those who had hepatitis B and 80 percent of patients with hepatitis C.

> My husband was laid off so I was nursing 16-hour shifts. That was in October. I got a needle-stick while I was taking care of a cancer patient

who was very jaundiced—orange like a pumpkin. In those days, you gave an injection and capped the needle with a safety cap. If you did it at the wrong angle, you got stuck. We had no sharps boxes where you could deposit the whole needle.

By November I was sick and in pain. I could only eat oatmeal and burnt toast. I thought it was my gallbladder, but it turned out to be hepatitis B.

Marie

In the U.S., hospital-based occupational health services test personnel for hepatitis B and vaccinate susceptible employees. More and more state laws and recent Department of Labor Occupational Safety & Health Administration (OSHA) directives now require the use of safe needle technology. Worldwide, unsafe injection practices cause an estimated 8 to 26 million hepatitis B cases a year. The World Health Organization and other partners have formed the Safe Injection Global Network (SIGN) to tackle the problem.

How do we treat people who have a needle-stick accident? First, doctors test them for the hepatitis B surface antibody. If the surface antibody is positive, they are immune and need no further treatment. If the surface antibody is negative, they are susceptible and should be given HBIG plus the hepatitis B vaccine as close as possible to the time of exposure.

Tattooing and Body Piercing

Tattooing and body piercing are ancient rites in many cultures. In this country, we're witnessing a recent surge of interest in "body art." The practice of tattooing is particularly common in the military and among gang members and prisoners. It's also becoming an accepted cosmetic practice.

Celebrities have popularized the trend. Comedian Roseanne and ex-husband Tom Arnold had each other's names tattooed on their backsides. Famous athletes have decorated their bodies, including Mike Peluso's tattoo of the Stanley Cup and Steve Everitt's bleeding dagger. Unfortunately, even the most benign-appearing tattooing may have its dark side (see Figure 3). Viral hepatitis, mainly hepatitis B, is the best documented infection transmitted by tattoos in the 20th century.

Here's a switch. I'm a tattoo artist, and last year I found out I have hepatitis C. I have antibodies to hepatitis B, too. My joints hurt so

FIGURE 3: HEPATITIS PATIENT WITH TATTOO

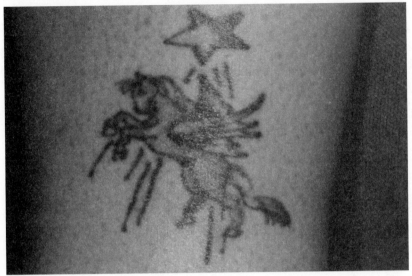

LEGEND 3: This seemingly innocuous tattoo may have been a source of transmission of hepatitis to this patient.

much, I can't work. I feel like I'm sliding down the evolutionary scale, because I can't move my opposable thumbs.

I'm sure I got hepatitis from a needle stick. Fifteen years ago, who wore gloves?

Peter

Nine percent of males and 1 percent of females in the United States get tattoos—with peak ages between 14 and 22. And tattoos are common in certain groups at high risk for hepatitis and other viral infections: intravenous drug abusers, gang members, prostitutes, and prisoners. In one study 65 percent of prisoners had tattoos.

This flag on my arm—I was young and in the Navy. What did I know? Now I'm told that there are certified tattoo artists, and if you go to someone reputable, everything is sterilized.

Well, too late for me. It wasn't like that in Hong Kong.

Jerry

Tattooing involves shaving the skin, placing ink on it, then pushing the ink through the skin with a needle gun. A small amount of bleeding is common. The problem is that sterilization techniques vary, and home-tattooing kits may contain inadequate methods for sterilization.

Body piercing of the earlobes, nose, lips, and other areas also breaks the skin. Therefore, the principles and risk of transmission of hepatitis B are the same as in tattooing.

Household Contact / Casual Contact

I raised four children while having hepatitis B. I don't know why my kids didn't get it. Now that I'm aware I have the virus, I tell everyone I know to get vaccinated, and I hope they do. I take reasonable precautions, but we can't live in plastic wrap!

The way I see it, those of us with hepatitis B need to be safe and responsible—and that is all we can do.

Thomas

People who live in close contact with those infected with hepatitis B are at risk. Household contact refers to people living in the same dwelling but who do not have sexual relations. The risk of household contacts acquiring hepatitis B is lower than with close personal contact, but there is still risk of transmission.

Talk to family members and explain why it's important to avoid sharing razor blades, nail clippers, scissors, and toothbrushes. These measures are just good hygiene; it's also sensible to bandage any cuts or abrasions and to safely dispose of menstrual pads and tampons.

In my clinical experience I have seen only one case where the transmission of hepatitis B occurred due to sharing sharp objects. In this case hepatitis B was transmitted from brother to sister because they commonly shared a shaving razor blade.

I found out my brother had hepatitis B when he was 18. My parents were ignorant about hepatitis. "Oh, he's fine," they said. "He'll be okay."

So when I flew back to my hometown for my grandmother's funeral, I stayed with my brother. I knew he had hepatitis B, but I didn't know it was contagious. I used his razor blade and nicked myself. I asked my dad if I could get sick from my brother, and he said no.

I was so tired that winter. A year later, I got pregnant and was screened for hepatitis B. I tested positive, but my DNA was undetectable. I'm a chronic carrier.

Perhaps I got it from my brother, but I found out I have other risk factors, too, because I've lived in developing countries. My biopsy didn't look good so maybe I had the virus for a long time—maybe even since birth.

Tammie

Casual contact refers to people in the workplace, school, and other organizations where there is no personal contact or the potential for sharing sharp objects and other hygienic utensils. Casual contacts are not at increased risk, and therefore neither HBIG nor vaccine is necessary.

Institutional Contact

People who live in institutional settings, such as residents of homes for the developmentally disabled and prison inmates, are at increased risk. Risk is related to poor hygienic practice and activities that increase the potential for blood-to-blood transmission. Testing of residents for susceptibility to hepatitis B infection and universal vaccination programs may eliminate this problem.

Organ Transplantation

Can a person get hepatitis B from a transplanted organ? Yes, if the donor tests positive for prior hepatitis B exposure. Organs from donors who are positive for hepatitis B surface antigen are not used for transplantation. However, organs from donors who test negative for hepatitis B surface antigen but positive for hepatitis B core antibody are used—although these organs are usually restricted to recipients with hepatitis B (see Chapter 9).

Can you, as a hepatitis B patient, donate an organ? Yes, if you lack surface antigen, and your only markers of hepatitis B are core or suface antibodies. Transplanting organs from core antibody donors into non-infected susceptible recipients can lead to infection of the recipient in 50 percent of cases. Transplant programs have protocols to reduce the risk of infection in those recipients. The organs most commonly used are the kidney and liver, but only if the liver shows no active disease or scarring.

How Can I Avoid Infecting Others?

My patients often inquire about protecting friends and family from the virus. Here are some common questions people ask:

Is it okay to kiss and hug my kids? Yes, you can kiss and hug your children, and they can kiss and hug you back. There is no data to suggest that you could infect your children by these actions.

Should I have members of my family tested for hepatitis B? Yes. There is definite risk of transmission to a sexual partner, spouse, and even other family members and household contacts. Once again, family members should be vaccinated.

Can I cook for my family? What if I cut myself while I'm preparing food? Certainly you can cook for your family. Even if you cut yourself and get blood in the food, it's unlikely that anyone eating the food will get hepatitis B. The enzymes in the digestive tract will destroy or inactivate the virus.

What if my child or friend eats food off my plate or uses my fork? You don't transmit hepatitis B by sharing drinks or food. Hepatitis B is transmitted by contaminated blood entering your bloodstream—not your stomach.

In some Asian cultures, caregivers pre-chew food for babies. It is hypothetically possible to transmit hepatitis B through saliva if the chewer and baby have mouth sores or bloody gums. Sharing of toothbrushes, towels, and anything else that might come in contact with blood or body fluids can also expose people to the same hypothetical risks. Even though these are not common or likely infection routes, it makes good common sense to avoid such behaviors for hygienic reasons.

My teenager borrowed my manicure scissors. Is that a problem? I recommend that you avoid sharing sharp instruments. There is a possibility that if your teenager cut herself on your scissors, she could inoculate herself with blood you might have left on the scissors. It's best to avoid sharing all sharp instruments, such as nail clippers, razor blades, toothbrushes, etc.

We've been married for 15 years. Is it safe to have sex? Yes, but be sure your partner is tested for hepatitis B. If the tests are negative, get your partner vaccinated. About 5 to 10 percent of sex partners will already have been exposed and formed protective antibodies. If not, they should be vaccinated.

What about French kissing? Oral sex? One of the most common questions I'm asked has to do with the risk of transmission during sexual activity. If you are involved in a stable, long-term relationship, your partner can be protected by vaccination and HBIG. I recommend that partners be informed of infection and preventive measures. Once partners take these measures and are immune, they are protected during all sexual activity, including French kissing and oral sex.

I'm single. What should I tell my dates? You have a trust issue to resolve that requires disclosing your hepatitis B infection. Place the disclosure in the context of knowing that your hepatitis B infection need not fracture or destroy an otherwise promising relationship. Infected people should notify their sexual partners and inform them that effective preventive measures are available: vaccination and HBIG.

Should I always use condoms? My advice is not to engage in sexual activity unless your partner is protected. However, we do understand that casual, spur-of-the-moment sexual encounters happen. In this situation latex condoms and safe sex practices may reduce—but not eliminate—the risk of transmission.

Can I have a baby? Nurse my baby? Yes. Current treatment of infants at the time of delivery can nearly eliminate the risk that babies will become infected. Once the babies are immune, they cannot be infected by any other exposure, including mother's milk. Even so, infants who are not immune and still susceptible to infection are not likely to get hepatitis B from breastfeeding. (For more information, see Chapter 12.)

Is it necessary to tell people like my dentist that I have hepatitis B? Yes. Patients should inform dentists and other health care professionals who need to perform invasive procedures or operations.

How do I clean up a blood spill? If you have gloves available, use them. If not, take precautions to prevent contact of the blood with your skin or any cuts, abrasions, sores, or wounds on your skin. Take a rag or paper cloth and wipe the spill. If household bleach is available, use diluted bleach at the site of the spill. Dispose of the rag or paper in a plastic bag, and throw it in the garbage. Wash your hands afterwards. The term "Universal Precautions" when dealing with potentially infectious matter means to wear gloves, avoid exposure to infection, and wash your hands.

What about biting? Spitting? Biting is a potential mode of transmission when the bite breaks the skin, allowing the virus to enter. Spit that gets in the eye or nose also can be a potential problem. Theoretically, the virus could pass through the mucous membrane of the eye or nose, but this is an unlikely scenario.

Can I play contact sports? When there is potential for bloody trauma, contact sports can result in the transmission of hepatitis B. A recent study in the *Archives of Internal Medicine* describes 11 cases of hepatitis B infection on a Japanese football team that were traced to a single player. With universal vaccination, this risk can be eliminated.

> *We learn geology the morning after the earthquake.*
>
> *Emerson*

Reference
[1] Alter, Harvey J., C. Conry-Cantilena, J. Melpolder, D. Tan, M. Van Raden, D. Herion, D. Lau, J.H. Hoofnagle, "Hepatitis C in Asymptomatic Blood Donors," *Hepatology* 1997; 26 (Suppl 1): 295-335.

4

LEARNING ABOUT YOUR LIVER: YOUR BODY'S CHEMICAL FACTORY

Liver Facts and Liver Disease Symptoms

from Oda al Higado (Ode to the Liver)[1]
by Pablo Neruda
. . . navigating
the hidden mysteries,
the alchemist's chamber
of life's microscopic,
echoic, inner oceans . . .

Translated by Herberto Morales and Will Hochman

IMAGINE A MACHINE that converts food into energy; stores nutrients, fats, and vitamins; makes proteins for blood plasma; and detoxifies poisons. Your liver does all this and more—much more. But no machine, no matter how powerful, is as versatile as your liver. Even if 75 percent of the liver's mass is taken away, it still functions. And it's the only internal organ that regenerates itself.

This chapter will discuss what the liver looks like, how it functions, and what happens to the liver when it's infected with hepatitis B— including ten warning signals your body sends you when liver function is compromised.

- Liver Facts from Mesopotamian to Modern Times
- A Look at Your Liver
    Appearance
    Under the Microscope
- How Your Liver Works
    Blood
    Bile
    Lymph
    Immune System
    Chemical Factory
    Bilirubin
    ALT, AST, GGT, Alkaline Phosphatase
    Albumin
    Clotting Factors
    Hormones
- Phases of Hepatitis B
    Phase I: Infection
    Phase II: Inflammation
    Phase III: Fibrosis
    Phase IV: Cirrhosis
- Ten Danger Signs of Liver Disease
    Early Warning Signs: #1–#2
        #1: Early Symptoms
        #2: Changes in Liver Functions
    Later Warning Signs of Cirrhosis: #3–#10
        Compensated Cirrhosis
        Decompensated Cirrhosis
        #3: Changes in the Appearance of the Skin: Jaundice, Spider Nevi (Telangiectasia), Palmar Erythema
        #4: Fluid Buildup: Ascites
        #5: Bleeding: Variceal Hemorrhage
        #6: Mental Confusion: Encephalopathy
        #7: Weight Loss

#8: Thinning of Bones (Osteoporosis) and Fractures
Metabolic Bone Disease
#9: Blood Clotting Problems: Coagulopathy
#10: Itching: Pruritus
- Beyond the Liver: Conditions Associated with Hepatitis B
  Kidney Damage: Membranous Nephropathy
  Inflammation of the Arteries: Polyarteritis Nodosa
  Hives: Urticaria
  Arthritis
  Inflammation of Skeletal Muscle: Myocytis
  Sjögren Syndrome
  Carditis
  Neuritis

Liver Facts from Mesopotamian to Modern Times

- Mesopotamians didn't know anatomy, but they could see that the liver seemed to be the collecting point for blood, the source of life. Archeologists have found 5,000-year-old Mesopotamian clay models of livers with markings that may have helped priests perform religious rites.
- In ancient cultures, animals were sacrificed before battle and their entrails were examined; a healthy blood-red liver was a good omen. Pale livers foretold defeat—an expression that has entered the English language with the term "lily-livered," meaning cowardly.
- In Greek mythology, Prometheus stole fire from the gods and gave it to mankind. Zeus punished him by chaining him to a rock in the mountains. Each day an eagle gnawed at his body, feasting on his liver. Because the liver has such great regenerating capacity, it grew back each night, subjecting Prometheus to an endless ordeal.
- In 1987, a granite sculpture of the liver was unveiled in Ferrol, Spain. The city's coroner, who doubled as the mayor, said that over the years he saw "hundreds of these organs tortured by cocktails, wine, tranquilizers, and other medications . . . but every day, the poor little liver is at work neutralizing and purifying everything we take in."[2] As the monument was dedicated, a local poet recited "Oda Al Higado" (Ode to the Liver) by the late Nobel prize-winner, Pablo Neruda.

A Look at Your Liver

Appearance. As a hepatologist, a doctor who studies livers, I sometimes forget that my patients usually don't have a clear idea of what this organ looks like.

> *When I was diagnosed with hepatitis, I had no idea what my liver did or even where it was located. I had this pain in my midsection. It felt like a muscle pain, but it seemed to get worse after meals. I thought maybe my liver was getting worse.*
>
> *Finally, I went to the doctor. "That's not your liver; it's the end of your esophagus," he said, pushing down. I gave a yelp. What I thought was pain due to my liver was pain due to gas!*
>
> *Janet*

Learning more about your liver can give you a greater feeling of control and reduce stress, so let's examine this organ—the largest one in your body. The liver weighs about three pounds in an adult male and sits in the upper right of the abdomen, protected by the rib cage (see Figure 4A).

If you've ever gone to the supermarket or butcher, you've seen animal livers. They give you a pretty good idea of what the human liver looks and feels like. Reddish-brown in color, it's shaped like a flattened football with two lobes. The larger lobe lies closest to your right side.

The liver is surrounded by vital organs: diaphragm and lungs above, kidney behind, intestine and colon below.

Major blood vessels serve as conduits to deliver blood to and from the liver. Your blood system transports food, oxygen, and waste. Because your liver is a central depot for so many body functions, it has the largest and most complex blood supply of any organ in the body. In fact, about 1.5 quarts of blood flow through the liver every minute.

Like other parts of your body, the liver has an artery to supply it with oxygenated blood (the hepatic artery via the abdominal aorta) and hepatic veins to take blood back to the heart. The hepatic veins join the inferior vena cava, the major vein just below the diaphragm.

In addition to the hepatic artery, the liver has a second source of blood, the portal vein. This vein is responsible for at least two-thirds of liver blood flow and delivers nutrients, medications, and toxins absorbed by the intestine to the liver for processing.

FIGURE 4A. ANATOMIC LOCATION OF THE LIVER IN HUMANS

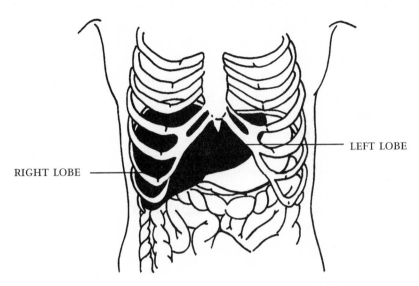

RIGHT LOBE

LEFT LOBE

LEGEND 4A: The liver is located in the right upper quadrant of the abdomen and is protected from external trauma by the rib cage.

Have you ever wondered why livers are a dull red color? It's because the portal vein transports nutrients to the liver in dark, deoxygenated blood.

Speaking of colors, your liver produces up to a quart a day of yellow-green bile, a liquid that looks like motor oil and breaks down fat in foods. Bile flows from the liver into the bile duct, which resembles the branches of a tree. The smallest branches are embedded in the liver while the common bile duct is the tree "trunk."

The common bile duct connects with the gallbladder (which stores bile and is attached to the underside of your liver) through the cystic duct. Then the bile duct continues through the pancreas, where it's joined by the pancreatic duct, and on to the upper intestine (duodenum).

Under the Microscope. Tiny units, called lobules, are the building blocks of your liver tissue. Each lobule is a spheroid structure and measures about 0.2 inches across. Under the microscope, you see flat sheets of cube-shaped liver cells (hepatocytes) fanning out from a tiny central vein. Blood flows in the spaces (sinusoids) between the liver cells.

Small branches of the hepatic artery (bringing oxygen from the heart) and the portal vein enter the lobule from the side and first deliver blood to the periphery of the lobule (portal area). Blood travels through the lobule toward its center, bathing the hepatocytes with nutrients, chemicals and toxins carried from the intestine. Medications that you take by mouth are also delivered to the liver in a similar fashion. Liver cells have special ways of extracting compounds from blood and metabolizing them—a topic I'll talk about in the next section.

The center of the lobule contains a very fine terminal branch of the hepatic vein. This vein then connects with other branches and "processed" blood flows through the hepatic veins to the inferior vena cava, returning to the heart.

In addition, each liver cell makes and secretes bile to its own tiny attached branch of the biliary system. The liver contains a whole network of these fine tubes that pipe bile to the bile duct and gallbladder.

How Your Liver Works

Knowing how the liver works will help you understand why things go wrong when a virus attacks it. Your liver affects your blood, bile, lymph, immune system, and chemical functions.

> I've had a smoldering hepatitis B infection for years and years. Then, although I didn't know it at the time, I got an acute attack of hepatitis A.
> My vision blurred. My hands shook. I ran a high fever. Then I became jaundiced, bloated, and confused. I had no clotting factors. My liver shut down, and my labs went off the charts. Weeks later, my bilirubin was 25—that's how bad it was.
>
> Al

Blood. The liver greatly influences the makeup of blood in your body. Blood is composed of plasma (a liquid), red cells, white cells, and platelets. When the liver is diseased, all of these blood components may be affected.

Do you know how your body tissues get oxygen? Red blood cells deliver it. Do you know why wounds clot? Platelets plug bleeding capillaries and vessels, and other clotting factors (proteins mainly synthesized by your liver) adhere to this platelet plug to solidify the clot. When you have an infection, white blood cells rush to the site as your first line of defense.

The liver receives blood from two sources: two-thirds from the portal vein (which comes from the intestine loaded with nutrients for the liver to process) and one-third from the hepatic artery. The hepatic artery, like all arteries, carries blood loaded with oxygen. About 15 percent of the blood pumped by the heart each minute runs through the liver.

As the liver becomes progressively injured, scar tissue builds up, making it difficult for blood from the portal vein and hepatic artery to flow through the liver. The blood tends to back up into other abdominal vessels and the spleen. As blood backs up in the spleen, the spleen enlarges. Cells become trapped and are destroyed—resulting in a decrease in platelets, red cells, and white cells.

Other factors also contribute to decreased blood counts in patients with liver disease. Patients with advanced disease develop nutritional or vitamin impairments, such as folate deficiency. Folate is an essential vitamin for normal blood formation by the bone marrow, and deficiency results in low red blood counts (anemia). Alcohol directly suppresses the function of the bone marrow, resulting in depressed counts of red cells, white cells, and platelets. Thrombopoeitin is a hormone made by the liver to stimulate the bone marrow to produce platelets. With advanced liver disease, thrombopoeitin production may decrease and further diminish platelet counts.

Bile. Did you know that cholesterol is an ingredient in bile? Your liver makes bile from water, electrolytes (sodium, potassium, chloride, and others), proteins, organic salts (bilirubin), and lipids (cholesterol, among others). The liver turns compounds that don't dissolve in water into water-soluble substances that are secreted into bile. Toxins (poisons) absorbed from the intestine also circulate in blood to the liver, which extracts, inactivates, and secretes them into bile. Many of the medications that you take by mouth are altered or processed by the liver.

Back to cholesterol. A normal part of our diets, it's made by several cells in our bodies. When too much cholesterol accumulates, cells may alter their functions and even die. If too much cholesterol builds up in blood vessels, you may get hardening of the arteries (atherosclerosis). If it builds up in bile, you may develop gallstones.

Prevention of these complications depends on eliminating excess cholesterol. Your liver is the only organ that breaks down cholesterol into bile acid, secretes it in bile, and removes it from your body for good.

What else does bile do? Simply put, bile helps you absorb fat and vitamins that are dissolved in fat (A, D, E, and K). When disease interrupts this cycle, your body has trouble digesting and absorbing fats and fat-soluble vitamins and getting rid of pigments and toxins. Processing of medications may also be impaired if your liver is severely damaged, and your doctor may need to adjust the doses of your medications.

Lymph. Your liver produces about a quart of lymph a day. Filtered from plasma, it's a protein-rich fluid composed mostly of water and electrolytes. Lymph travels through channels next to the portal vein and joins other major lymph channels in the abdomen. Eventually, the lymph is dumped into the bloodstream.

Any kind of disruption, whether it's disease or congestion of the lymph channels, may mean that large amounts of lymph spill into the abdomen. Although this rarely happens, it may be one reason for swelling of the abdomen due to fluid (ascites).

Immune System. Here's a mouthful: lymphocytes, plasma cells, macrophages, fibroblasts, dendritic cells, and polymorphonuclear leucocytes. All types of immune cells, including these, are found in the liver. In fact, the liver is one of the major lymphoid organs of the immune system.

The immune cells in the liver protect against infections or toxins, but may also, in certain diseases, cause liver injury. In hepatitis B, for example, the virus alone may cause little, if any, liver damage. Inflammation caused by the immune response to the virus produces most of the damage.

Chemical Factory. Your liver acts as a chemical powerhouse—building the substances you need for life and neutralizing or safely dumping harmful material. In fact, your liver performs more than 500 complex chemical functions!

I hope you're beginning to see that your liver works overtime to help and protect you. Take your digestive system, for instance. The liver stores nutrients, then sends them out to the parts of your body that need them.

When you eat carbohydrates (potatoes, pasta, and other starches), your body breaks them down into glucose. You need glucose for energy, but because of your liver, you don't have to eat carbohydrates all day long. Instead, the liver stores glucose as glycogen. When you need a burst of energy, your liver turns glycogen back into glucose and sends it through the bloodstream to your body.

Some of the fats you eat build new cells. The liver sends extra fat into the blood and, eventually, your body stores it as fat cells (adipose tissue). If you run out of carbohydrates, the fat stored in your liver becomes a major source of body fuel.

Protein you eat is broken down in your gut into amino acids, which are absorbed and distributed via the bloodstream to your liver and body. Cells use the amino acids to make new proteins or burn the amino acids for fuel. Proteins made by the liver regulate your clotting system, transport fat and nutrients throughout your body, control hormone levels, and maintain your blood volume.

Bilirubin. Bilirubin is the yellow pigment responsible for jaundice. When red blood cells in your body break down, they release hemoglobin—a molecule that carries oxygen to your tissues.

Enzymes are proteins that make specific chemical reactions take place. One of these enzymes, called heme oxygenase, occurs in bone marrow and liver cells. It converts heme, the major component of hemoglobin, into bilirubin. The liver then removes the bilirubin from your blood and turns it into a water-soluble form that is excreted into bile.

Normally, the amount of bilirubin produced approximates the rate of red blood cell breakdown. Bilirubin levels rise when something goes wrong, such as the breakdown of too many red blood cells, the development of liver disease (such as hepatitis), a defect in liver metabolism, or a blockage of the bile system. Bilirubin accumulates in tissues, causing your skin and the white part of your eyes (sclerae) to turn yellow.

ALT (SGPT), AST (SGOT), GGT, Alkaline Phosphatase. Your liver creates all of these enzymes. When liver cells are injured, the enzymes escape and enter the bloodstream. If small numbers of cells are affected, there may be little or no increase in plasma levels of enzymes. When large numbers of liver cells are injured or die, the levels of these enzymes in plasma increase markedly.

Enzyme tests roughly reflect the level of ongoing injury, but they don't indicate how your liver is actually functioning. To do that, you need to look at the tests that measure your liver's ability to build and synthesize (albumin, clotting factors) or to excrete (bilirubin).

Albumin. The liver makes this protein. It is vital for maintaining body fluid balance, especially the volume of plasma in your blood.

Although albumin levels in plasma may be affected by other disorders, in liver disease the level of serum albumin is a good marker of your liver's ability to produce proteins. A sustained decrease below the normal range is one of the first signs of advancing liver disease.

Clotting Factors. The liver also makes many proteins that help the blood to clot. In contrast to albumin, which stays a long time in plasma, clotting factors have a relatively short survival period. Therefore, the liver must constantly work to produce enough coagulation factors to maintain normal clotting.

When the liver is injured and can't make clotting factors, plasma levels drop within one or two days. Soon patients notice that they're bruising or bleeding easily even after minor bumps and injuries. If liver failure occurs, patients may hemorrhage and often require plasma and blood transfusions.

Hormones. In late stages of liver disease (cirrhotic phase), patients may experience hormonal imbalances, including altered ovulation or gonadal function and impairment of the pituitary gland (the main hormone control center). For example, men with cirrhosis often develop distressing enlargement of their breasts. Women may stop having menstrual periods. Disordered regulation of pituitary hormones may interrupt normal body functions, such as sleep-wake cycle, appetite, and body temperature.

I'm going to have a discussion with my doctors. A side effect of the anti-depressant I'm taking is low libido function. I'd like to know if it's that or the hepatitis B. I'm waiting for a transplant so I don't know if it's due to advanced liver disease or the medicine.

Robert

The men in my family have a history of larger than normal breasts, but my breasts seemed to be getting even bigger. I started getting lumps and hardness, especially in the nipple area. It's inflamed and uncomfortable.

My doctor sent me for a mammogram. It was negative. He said the enlargement was from one of the meds I was taking for edema, and he cut the dosage back. The swelling comes and goes, but it never goes away; the breasts remain. That's just cosmetic. The liver is the problem.

Ed

Phases of Hepatitis B

Figure 4B diagrams the consequences of hepatitis B infection. Hepatitis B infection and disease may be divided into four overlapping phases:

    I. Infection
   II. Inflammation
  III. Fibrosis
  IV. Cirrhosis

Phase I: Infection. When the hepatitis B virus gets into the bloodstream, it attaches to liver cells, enters them, and starts to reproduce. The new virus, made within the infected liver cell, exits into the bloodstream where it attaches to and infects another liver cell. This process allows the infection to spread through the liver.

FIGURE 4B. CONSEQUENCES OF HBV INFECTION

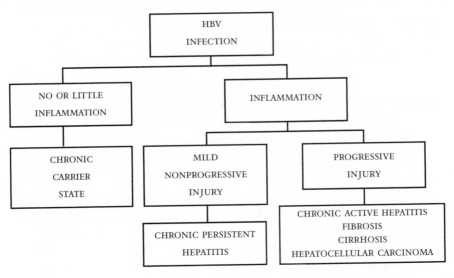

LEGEND 4B: Potential consequences of hepatitis B infection are shown. Some patients develop no or very little inflammation and co-exist with hepatitis B in a chronic carrier state. Others experience variable degrees of inflammation and liver damage. In the most severe cases, scarring becomes severe, resulting in cirrhosis or liver cancer (hepatocellular carcinoma—hepatoma).

Phase II: Inflammation. In this phase, liver inflammation (hepatitis) develops. Under the microscope, most liver cells appear relatively normal and uninjured. But in some areas there is liver cell injury and death. Inflammation in the liver is characterized by the presence of specific immune cells called lymphocytes. Lymphocytes are recruited to the liver to attempt to eliminate hepatitis B. However, they also release chemicals that damage liver cells and contribute to the liver injury.

In many cases, the initial acute phase of hepatitis B is mild in terms of symptoms. Many people don't realize they've had a first attack, and one percent or less experience sudden, severe (fulminant) liver failure due to the virus. About one-third of patients with acute infection develop jaundice.

Phase III: Fibrosis. Fibrosis, scar tissue, is a consequence of chronic infection and inflammation. Remember, only 5 to 10 percent of acutely infected adults develop chronic infection. If your liver biopsy shows significant fibrosis, it usually means you've had hepatitis B for several years.

Phase IV: Cirrhosis. When fibrosis increases, the fourth stage, cirrhosis, appears. With cirrhosis, the fibrosis is so severe that it affects how the liver functions and grossly distorts the architecture and blood flow of the liver.

Ten Danger Signs of Liver Disease

Warning symptoms fall into two categories: early and late. The liver sends few early warning signs. It's such a large organ with great reserve that most people can lose three-quarters of their liver without any change in function or development of symptoms.

In early hepatitis B, even though the liver is damaged, patients may have no symptoms. Symptoms early in the course of hepatitis B, such as muscle aches and headaches, are due to the virus itself and not to liver failure. Later in the course of hepatitis B, liver function diminishes and warning signs of advanced liver disease appear.

EARLY WARNING SIGNS: #1–#2

#1: Early Symptoms.

At our hepatitis support group, we compared notes. It turned out that four of us often experienced a tender, achy feeling on our right sides. Doctors had dismissed the symptom by saying the liver didn't feel pain—not to worry. But of course, we did.

So at my next medical appointment, I brought up the mystery symptom and got an answer. The liver doesn't feel pain, but the membrane around the liver and the liver itself may react to the inflammation from hepatitis.

I reported back to the group, and we all relaxed. Nothing had changed, but the simple explanation helped. It kept us from imagining that we were sliding into liver failure.

Hedy

Many people with hepatitis B, especially in the early phases, tell me they have no symptoms. I find, however, that if I question them closely, they complain of fatigue, feel less energetic, and are unable to work at their usual high level. Typically, appetite and weight are unaffected, but occasionally some patients report nausea and lack of appetite and so have difficulty maintaining their weight.

No one knows why these common symptoms occur. Some researchers think they're due to the viral infection itself, while others feel that the ongoing liver injury releases substances into the blood that produce these effects.

In my experience, these symptoms rarely, if at all, correspond to the severity of the disease. Some of my patients suffer extreme fatigue but have little injury to their livers, while others with aggressive hepatitis and cirrhosis may have no symptoms at all.

#2: Changes in Liver Functions. If you have hepatitis B, you need close medical supervision. Current recommendations call for an annual physical exam and liver blood tests every six months. Changes in blood tests usually pick up the first sign of deteriorating liver function.

At later stages of disease, albumin may decrease, bilirubin may rise, and prothrombin (a protein involved in blood clotting) time may increase. These changes occur because the liver is becoming less able to make its usual quota of substances the body needs. Another change that occurs is enlargement of the spleen. Platelets, white blood cells, and even red blood cells may drop because the enlarged spleen traps and destroys these cells. In my experience, a progressive buildup of fluid in the ankles and a low level of sodium in the blood are also common. These danger signs correlate with the cirrhotic stage. They indicate that the liver is less able to keep up with the amount of injury and often precede more serious symptoms of liver failure.

LATER WARNING SIGNS OF CIRRHOSIS: #3–#10

What does cirrhosis mean? Cirrhosis simply means the hardening of the liver due to a buildup of scar tissue and formation of nodules.

Compensated Cirrhosis. Patients who have early-stage cirrhosis, also known as compensated cirrhosis, may not have any symptoms or laboratory test abnormalities.

Decompensated Cirrhosis. Late-stage cirrhosis, or decompensated cirrhosis, is characterized by abnormalities in blood tests, complications (some of which are life threatening), and limited survival. Patients with any or all of the following signs may be potential candidates for a liver transplant.

#3: Changes in the Appearance of the Skin: Jaundice, Spider Nevi (Telangiectasia), Palmar Erythema.

Jaundice. Jaundice is the yellowing of the skin and whites of the eyes. It is due to an accumulation of the pigment bilirubin in these areas. Jaundice commonly occurs in patients with chronic hepatitis B when the liver disease is advanced and the hepatitis flares. In some cases, jaundice may disappear when the flare resolves.

> I got paged at work. "Something is wrong with me," John said. "Get over here." I raced home. He had what we thought was the flu, but I took one look at him and thought, oh my gosh, we're in trouble. I'm seeing an orange pumpkin here.
>
> I drove to the hospital like a bat out of hell. He was changing right before my eyes.
>
> *Marion*

Spider Nevi (Telangiectasia). Spider nevi are red spots, usually on the upper body and face. If you look at the spots closely, you will see a central red area with fine red lines emanating outward. These "spiders" are actually a collection of very small blood vessels caused by hormonal imbalance due to cirrhosis. The spiders disappear after transplantation.

Palmar Erythema. Palmar erythema is a reddening of the fleshy part of the palms of the hands. The condition occurs when blood vessels dilate because of hormonal imbalance due to cirrhosis. Palmar erythema and spider nevi often occur simultaneously.

#4: Fluid Buildup: Ascites. Ascites means that fluid builds up in the abdomen, so that the belly swells. Liver disease is the most common cause of ascites.

> *My stomach is a bit bloated, but I look like a regular guy. You wouldn't think I was so sick.*
>
> *Jerry*

> *I called my son and said, "I don't feel so good." My feet and ankles were swollen. My belly was getting big. I was a mess.*
>
> *They put me in the hospital. It was like I was going in for last rites. The doctor told my son I had two weeks left to live. Then they tapped me and got a pint of liquid out. They couldn't get it all even though they tried twice. But I got to go home, and I went on lamivudine. I've been on it ever since.*
>
> *Elizabeth*

Physicians must remove and analyze the fluid to exclude other causes. To remove fluid the physician performs a paracentesis, which involves placing a needle through the abdominal wall and drawing out the fluid for a culture, cell count, biochemical tests, and a microscopic examination. If the ascites is due to liver disease, the fluid will be clear, yellow, uninfected, and have a low cell count.

More than one problem, however, may be involved. Sometimes patients have a bacterial infection in the ascites (spontaneous bacterial peritonitis). In these cases, there are other signs of infection: fever, high white blood count, abdominal pain. It's important to recognize this condition right away and treat it early with antibiotics. We now have many treatments for ascites, including diuretics (drugs that increase the amount of urine excreted), paracentesis (drawing off fluid), or shunts (tubes that redirect the liquid), such as peritoneovenous shunts and transjugular intrahepatic portal-systemic shunts.

Muscle cramps are a common problem in patients with advanced liver disease. In particular, patients with ascites who are treated with diuretics commonly complain of severe cramping. This type of cramping may respond to reducing diuretics or administering magnesium, calcium, or possibly zinc.

Ascites is a serious warning sign of very advanced liver disease, and most patients with ascites will require a liver transplant for prolonged survival.

#5: Bleeding: Variceal Hemorrhage. The most dramatic and urgent complication of advanced liver disease is variceal hemorrhage. "Variceal" refers to varices, which are abnormally distended or swollen veins usually located in the esophagus, and "hemorrhage," of course, means bleeding.

Patients vomit large quantities of red blood, show signs of altered mental status, and have very low blood pressure. By the time they get to the emergency room, they may be in shock.

I didn't have a clue that I was sick. I was working full time as a florist, and I walked to and from work. One day I thought I had the flu so I stayed home—the first time in four-and-a-half years—because my stomach was upset. The next day I went back to work. By mid-afternoon I was nauseous and weak. My husband had to come get me.

By midnight I was vomiting blood. We lived in the mountains, and a helicopter carried me to the hospital. The wind was howling—blowing 80 miles per hour, and the chopper was rocking back and forth.

At the hospital, the doctor told me I had hepatitis B and I might be a candidate for a liver transplant!

Susan

My husband was complaining that he didn't feel good. He had diarrhea-like symptoms—black stool—for a month. We didn't know that meant bleeding.

Finally, I made an appointment with the doctor for him. I got a call from the hospital emergency room. Joe had lost so much blood, he was anemic. His belly was swollen. He was retaining water. They did a scope. The veins down his throat, his esophagus, were huge and filled with blood. These were all symptoms of advanced liver disease, but we didn't know.

Maria

It's urgent to get to an emergency medical facility when there's any sign of bleeding from the upper gastrointestinal tract. Variceal bleeding may be indicated by vomiting red blood, the passage of loose, dark, tarry feces, or the passage of a large amount of red blood through the rectum.

Doctors first must find the source of the bleeding before they can treat the problem. They insert a slender tube (endoscope) down the patient's throat to diagnose the cause or source of the bleed. Endoscopists have two treatments available: tying the bleeding veins with bands (ligation) or injecting a chemical into the vein to make it clot (sclerotherapy). Both therapies work well to control the initial bleed. But to eradicate the varices and avoid later hemorrhages, outpatient treatments must be repeated—usually two or three times.

Doctors may also give medications such as somatostatin, vasopressin, nitroglycerin, and plasma products to control the bleeding. Sometimes propranolol or related medicines are given to lower the risk of a rebleed.

Occasionally, varices are also found in the stomach, duodenum, intestine, and colon. It's harder to manage varices in these locations with endoscopic treatment. Doctors often will treat bleeding from these varices with either a surgical shunt (a tube that redirects the blood) or TIPS. Surgical shunts require major abdominal surgery and connect one of the portal veins to veins that bypass the liver (systemic veins).

TIPS is short for transjugular intrahepatic portal-systemic shunt. Radiologists put the TIPS in place, avoiding the need for risky abdominal surgery that might compromise a later liver transplant.

First, the radiologist places a catheter through a vein in the neck, then into the liver via the hepatic veins. A needle goes through this catheter into the liver and punctures a main branch of the portal vein. Once the portal vein and hepatic veins are connected, the radiologist dilates the tract and places an expandable cylindrical wire-mesh shunt across the liver to maintain the connection. When the shunt is in place, it relieves the back pressure on the portal veins, varices collapse, and the risk of further hemorrhage is greatly reduced.

Transplant surgeons welcome TIPS because it doesn't interfere with their surgery. However, occasionally, TIPS migrate into the portal vein and complicate a transplant operation, so most transplant doctors prefer that TIPS be placed by radiologists with a high level of experience with the procedure.

#6: Mental Confusion: Portal-Systemic Encephalopathy. The liver conducts many metabolic functions, including clearing or detoxifying the blood of harmful substances. When the liver fails, these substances may build up to toxic levels and impair the function of other organs, such as the brain.

> *It's wild. I can feel it coming on. I get a panicky feeling, a scared feeling. Then it comes on.*
>
> *I don't know who I am or where I'm at. It's strange. I might have it for hours or all night long. My wife tells me I say I want the dogs to come inside—and we haven't had dogs for 20 years.*
>
> *Chris*

The brain reacts to altered liver functions, so patients with advanced liver disease commonly note changes in their mental abilities. These changes range from slight changes, such as decline in memory or reduced ability to perform complex calculations, to more severe changes, such as confusion, disorientation, blackout spells, or even coma.

It helps to understand four features of encephalopathy: (1) It is usually brought on by some other problem, such as gastrointestinal bleeding, infection, or electrolyte imbalance. (2) It's a completely reversible condition. (3) Effective medical therapy exists [lactulose (a non-absorbable carbohydrate), neomycin (an antibiotic), a protein-restricted diet]. Early therapy may prevent the patient from lapsing into more advanced stages, such as coma. (4) A successful liver transplant completely reverses the condition.

This means that a patient experiencing encephalopathy must get urgent medical attention and evaluation, be treated promptly, and be considered for liver transplantation.

#7: Weight Loss. Because the liver acts as your body's metabolic factory and energy storehouse, advancing liver disease affects your nutrition. That's why your doctor looks for weight loss.

> *After I got out of the hospital for the ascites, I was a mess. At home I went from 205 to 160 pounds in a month! I looked like a bloody old skeleton. I was scaring myself.*
>
> *Gary*

I'm getting worried about my continuous weight loss. Today I was wearing a pair of trousers, which were too tight when they were made for me back in 1985. They fell off me as I climbed the stairs! Now that's weight loss.

Steven

Patients need to eat an appropriate amount of calories. And because patients often are on a sodium restriction for ascites and a protein restriction for encephalopathy, that can be hard to do. I usually recommend supplements and a visit to a dietician.

Blood tests detect nutritional deficiencies. People with liver disease, for example, may have fat-soluble vitamin deficiencies (A, D, E, K) that can be at least partially corrected with oral supplements. I prefer retinyl palmitate (Vitamin A), Calderol® (Vitamin D-25-OH), tocopherol polyethylene glycol solution or TPGS (Vitamin E), and Mephyton® (Vitamin K). The TPGS formulation of Vitamin E is an emulsified liquid that also aids the absorption of A, D, and K. A simple way to think of TPGS is that it's artificial bile. I recommend that all the fat-soluble vitamins be taken with the TPGS to improve absorption.

#8: Thinning of Bones (Osteoporosis) and Fractures: Metabolic Bone Disease. Did you know that as liver disease progresses, bone loss may accelerate? Bone loss is frequently observed in patients with advanced hepatitis B, especially those receiving steroid medication for other conditions.

My husband was holding a ladder, and I went up two steps. He said not to go higher, but I did. On the third step I fell—right on my arm. I broke the top of the bone that goes to the shoulder.

I'm only in my 40s so I think I broke it because of my cirrhosis. And I was black and blue all over because my blood clotting time is off.

Laura

First, the doctor must exclude other causes of bone loss, such as Vitamin D deficiency or hyperparathyroidism. Typically, patients with bone disease and fractures due to end-stage liver disease simply have a condition called osteopenia, which does not respond well to Vitamin D, calcium, or fluoride. Recent studies suggest that a new drug, alendronate, may be of some benefit. To complicate matters, post-transplant use of steroids and the relative inactivity after surgery can make the bones more brittle. Most transplant centers now taper steroids sharply and encourage early ambulation to lower the risk of fractures.

#9: Blood Clotting Problems: Coagulopathy. People with end-stage liver disease have multiple defects in their blood clotting system that put them at risk for bleeding and hemorrhage.

> *On our vacation, the roots of my teeth snapped off. I looked pretty funny with two front teeth gone. I told the dentist I had advanced hepatitis B, and he said, "You'll bleed to death if I do dental surgery." But I told him to go ahead anyway—and I damn near did.*
>
> *We went out for dinner, and I was talking to my son-in-law, when all of a sudden I had a mouthful of blood.*
>
> *Saul*

Coagulation proteins and platelet counts drop to such low levels that even minor trauma to skin, gums, lips, or extremities causes marked bruising or prolonged oozing of blood. Major trauma, such as surgery, can result in excessive bleeding. In many cases your doctor may be able to administer clotting factors to reduce your risk of bleeding from these procedures. In addition, the spleen often holds and destroys platelets, reducing the body's other major clotting aid. If severe clotting disturbances develop, it's an ominous sign of advanced liver disease and means immediate consideration for a transplant.

#10: Itching: Pruritus. Constant itching, day and night, may torment patients with severe jaundice or advanced liver disease. It's caused by a buildup of substances in the skin that are normally cleared by the liver, and it's not associated with hives or rashes (except what people get from scratching). Although generalized, itching may be peculiarly localized to the palms of the hands, soles of the feet, inside the mouth, and the external ear canal.

> *That itching! I wake up in the middle of the night, itching and scratching. And you don't even know you've been doing it for an hour.*
>
> *Janice*

The creams don't work, but someone in my support group told me to use cornstarch. So now I bathe, dry myself off, and apply the cornstarch. I've done it three times so far, and it helps.

Bernie

The pruritus of liver disease does not respond to antihistamines, skin lotions, and creams, but improves with the use of medicines that promote bile flow, such as ursodeoxycholate, or that bind and inactivate substances in the intestine, such as cholestyramine.

Recent studies suggest that pruritus may be related to naturally occurring morphine-like compounds that build up in the patient and may respond to medications that block morphine effects (naloxone, naltrexone).

Some patients have severe, incapacitating pruritus that can't be helped by any of the therapies mentioned. A liver transplant successfully treats the condition.

Beyond the Liver: Conditions Associated with Hepatitis B

The ten danger signs of advanced liver disease and cirrhosis are common to all forms of liver disease, including hepatitis B. In addition, hepatitis B patients may find themselves dealing with other conditions associated with the virus. These conditions are called extra-hepatic (non-liver) manifestations of hepatitis B.

Although the hepatitis B virus primarily targets the liver, other organs and body tissues can be damaged. One cause of these injuries is due to an activated immune system directed against hepatitis B and its proteins. In the liver, the proteins of hepatitis B travel to the surface of the liver cells where they interact with cells of the immune system. The immune cells try to eliminate the hepatitis B (foreign protein). This reaction leads to liver cell damage.

In other parts of the body, the immune reaction is different. Most of your other body cells don't harbor the virus. Instead, your blood contains the virus, and the immune response is against the virus circulating in your blood.

A number of reactions can occur. One immune reaction involves antibody formation. The antibodies that form bind the virus or proteins of the virus and form immune complexes. The immune complexes are bulky, and they tend to deposit in very small blood vessels of the circulation, called capillaries. Once this occurs, the tissues can become inflamed, and other immune reactions (such as skin rashes) can occur. Common organs and tissues involved with these reactions include the kidney, blood vessels, muscle, and nerve tissue.

The two major extra-hepatic conditions that may arise in patients with chronic hepatitis B are kidney damage and polyarteritis nodosa. Rarely seen conditions include muscle damage (myocytis), Sjögren syndrome, cardiac injury (carditis), and neurologic injury (neuritis).

Kidney Damage: Membranous Nephropathy. A specific type of kidney damage, called membranous nephropathy, can occur when immune complexes containing the hepatitis B virus lodge in the kidney and cause inflammation. At first, there may be no symptoms. It's often detected when a routine urinalysis shows protein in the urine. As more protein is lost in urine, the blood albumin may decrease, and patients may notice swelling from fluid buildup in the ankles or abdomen. Progressive damage can lead to kidney failure. Membranous nephropathy, complicating hepatitis B, may respond to treatment with interferon (see Chapter 8).

Patients at greatest risk for this complication are those who have had hepatitis B for many years, usually decades. For this reason, patients who acquired the infection at birth—such as some immigrants from Southeast Asia, China and Africa—are at highest risk.

Many patients with this form of kidney damage may have little or no evidence of liver damage. Kidney damage in adults tends to be progressive, but in children it may resolve spontaneously (see Chapter 12).

Inflammation of the Arteries: Polyarteritis Nodosa. Polyarteritis nodosa, an inflammation of the body's medium-size arteries, is a serious complication of chronic hepatitis B that can lead to organ damage, severe medical illness, and even death. The inflammation weakens the arterial walls, thinning them and producing aneurysms. Polyarteritis nodosa is most commonly found in the arteries supplying blood to the intestines, liver, and kidneys. Both adult and pediatric patients are at risk, but those at greatest risk have had hepatitis B for many years.

The most common symptoms or clinical features are abdominal pain, neurological signs (seizures, leg weakness, attacks of blindness, and other stroke-like features), hypertension (high blood pressure), muscle and joint pain, cardiac inflammation, skin rash (including hives), and kidney disease. Please note that most cases of hives in patients with chronic hepatitis are not due to polyarteritis nodosa (see next section).

We use two strategies to treat polyarteritis nodosa. Because the inflammation is mediated by your immune system, one approach is to suppress the immune system using steroids and azathioprine (a nucleoside analogue). This treatment decreases inflammation and injury due to the immune reaction but favors ongoing replication of hepatitis B. The second approach is to use antiviral strategies to eradicate infection (see Chapter 8). Current treatment often combines these two approaches.

Hives: Urticaria. Hives due to hepatitis B typically occur at any time in the course of active hepatitis B infection. They develop as a consequence of the immune response to hepatitis B viral proteins, such as the hepatitis B surface antigen.

> *Suddenly I noticed that I was sensitive to cold. I almost couldn't go out in the winter because wherever my clothing got cold and rubbed against my skin, like at my waist and hips, I'd get welts.*
>
> *If I went swimming, when I got out of the pool the water evaporated on my skin. I'd feel cold, and then I'd see these hives. They really swelled and itched for about 15 minutes. Then I'd feel okay, and they'd disappear.*
>
> *As the virus in my system started going away, the symptoms diminished. But I still have it—just slightly.*
>
> *Bruce*

There are two main time periods for the occurrence of hives: (1) before the initial attack of acute hepatitis and (2) later, in patients who develop chronic infection. Hepatitis B circulates in the blood after infection but before liver damage occurs. The immune reaction to the circulating virus can cause an illness characterized by hives, joint pain and swelling, fever, and other flu-like symptoms. Called serum sickness, this illness typically clears spontaneously before the onset of liver damage. When hives occur later, in chronic infection, they tend to wax and wane in relation to viral replication and are sometimes associated with joint symptoms and fever.

Arthritis. Arthritis due to hepatitis B is also an immune complex disease. Joints can become painful, red, and swollen, but rarely do we see evidence of joint destruction. Symptoms may be relieved by anti-inflammatory drugs. Many of the older non-steroidal anti-inflammatory medicines, such as aspirin, ibuprofen, and naproxen irritate the stomach and can cause gastrointestinal bleeding. Newer agents, called COX-2 inhibitors (celecoxib, rofecoxib), suppress the inflammation without damaging the gastrointestinal tract and are currently preferred.

> *I had a big flare, and all of a sudden I felt like Job. I got arthritis in my right shoulder with limited range of motion. I couldn't swing my arm around. The next morning I woke up with arthritis in my left shoulder. I had this for six months, but the symptoms gradually diminished as the virus started going away.*
>
> *Of course, I got depressed. I've always been borderline, but this pushed me over the edge.*
>
> *Jerry*

Inflammation of Skeletal Muscle: Myocytis. Myocytis is inflammation and damage of skeletal muscle. Symptoms include muscle pain and weakness. Blood tests of patients with myocytis show elevations of muscle enzymes, such as creatine phosphokinase or aldolase. Treatment is similar to therapies used for arthritis.

Sjögren Syndrome. Sjögren syndrome is dryness of the eyes and mucous membranes of the mouth. It is caused by inflammation and damage to glands that secrete fluid and mucin (a protein in mucous secretions). The two main glands damaged are lacrimal glands that make tears and salivary glands that make saliva. Treatment for dry eyes includes the use of artificial tears and for dry mouth, lozenges to stimulate saliva production.

Carditis. Carditis is inflammation and damage to heart muscle cells. When severe, the damage can lead to poor heart function and heart failure. Treatment includes anti-inflammatory drugs and medicine to control heart failure. Treatment is directed at controlling the hepatitis B infection.

Neuritis. Neuritis is inflammation and damage to peripheral nerves. Symptoms are usually limited to lower extremities and can include pain, numbness, tingling, and weakness. Treatment is directed at controlling the hepatitis B infection and uses anti-inflammatory medicines. In some cases, the nerve damage can progress and become permanent.

In summary, extra-hepatic manifestations occur often in patients with hepatitis B. The two primary goals of treatment for these extra-hepatic manifestations are suppressing inflammation and damage and, of course, eliminating the hepatitis B infection.

. . .

Reading this list of what can go wrong with your liver anticipates the worst that can happen. Remember that a majority of the people who develop chronic hepatitis B may not progress to cirrhosis. Nevertheless, it's important to know what the symptoms are, so you can report any changes promptly to your physician.

In the next chapters, we'll take a look at ways you can help your liver with healthy eating habits and stress-reduction techniques. I'll contribute a medical perspective, we'll hear from experts who specialize in these areas, and we'll listen to patients as they share their personal stories.

The beginning of health is to know the disease.

Miguel de Cervantes

References
1 Pablo Neruda. *Nuevas Odas Elementales.* Buenos Aires: Editorial Losada, p. 76-80.
2 "Sculpture in Spain Salutes the 'Silent, Unselfish' Liver," *Austin American-Statesman*, 28 June 1987:A2.

5

TAKING CARE OF
YOURSELF
NUTRITIONALLY

Guidelines for Healthy
Nutrition in Liver Disease

*At first, when I was still in shock over the diagnosis of chronic hep-
atitis, I was too scared to try interferon. So I decided to do all I could with
"natural" methods. I went to two dieticians who recommended a low-fat
diet to take a load off my liver. They also advocated intravenous vitamin
C and coffee enemas, which turned me off.*

*Then I saw a naturopath. He restricted my diet in so many ways, I
lost ten pounds. I never looked so good! But I still felt tired, so I consulted a nutritionist. She told me to keep a food journal, which made it
possible for us to review my diet and my eating patterns.*

*I had been skimping on protein because I thought that would help
my liver. Turns out that protein restriction is only for people in end-stage
liver disease who are mentally confused. So she suggested I eat enough
protein but divide my portions into smaller amounts throughout the day.
I followed her suggestions and started to feel more energy.*

Looking back, I can see what I was trying to do—control what I could in a world that suddenly seemed so out of control. I might not be able to stop the virus, but I could decide what I put into my body.

After a while, I found that all the junk food I used to love didn't taste so good anymore. I gave up the artificially sweet stuff I used to eat. Now a crisp apple or some strawberries flood my mouth with natural flavor. It's ironic, but learning I was ill made me "healthier."

Hedy

MANY PEOPLE, when they discover they have hepatitis B, become interested in improving their general health through good nutrition. I encourage patients to learn how to eat in a healthier way, but to avoid crash diets and food fads that promise more than they can deliver.

Caution: Always check with your doctor before making major changes in your diet or taking over-the-counter supplements and vitamins. Some seemingly harmless substances can injure your liver.

In the early, noncirrhotic stages of hepatitis B, people can maintain normal nutrition if they eat a well-balanced diet. It's rare for a doctor to recommend supplements beyond one multivitamin a day. However, as the disease progresses, malnutrition and vitamin deficiencies may develop.

Nutritional therapy includes the following goals:

- to maintain the appropriate balance between the calories you take in and the calories your body requires
- to avoid malnutrition or deficiencies in specific nutrients
- to use appropriate supplementation when needed

In this chapter, I'll discuss some general nutritional concepts, what happens when liver disease affects your nutrition, and some specific deficiencies and their treatments:

- Nutritional Overview
  Ideal Body Weight
  Normal Diet
- Nutrition and the Liver
  Carbohydrate Metabolism
  Protein Metabolism
  Fat Metabolism

> *Bile*
> *Vitamins*
- Nutritional Needs for Hepatitis B Patients without Cirrhosis
  > *Caloric Requirements*
  > *Vitamin Supplements*
  > *Nutritional (Herbal) Therapies*
  > *Herbs Harmful to the Liver*
  > *Nutrition Tips from Patients*
- Nutritional Needs for Hepatitis B Patients with Cirrhosis
  > *Caloric Requirements*
  > *Protein Restriction*
  > *Vitamin Supplements*
  > *Mineral Supplements*
  > *Salt and Fluid Restriction*

Nutritional Overview

The liver is your body's major digestive organ. When the liver receives nutrients from the intestines, it metabolizes,* packages, stores, and sends the nutrients to other organs where they are used for energy. Your liver's major nutritional jobs include:

- metabolizing carbohydrates, proteins, and fat for energy
- assimilating and storing vitamins
- manufacturing bile to aid in digestion and absorption of fats
- filtering and destroying toxins (including alcohol and drugs)

Ideal Body Weight. Most people worry about their weight, with good reason. One in three American adults is overweight, a statistic that's up from one in four only a decade ago. With advanced liver disease, however, a major concern is the opposite problem, nutritional wasting.

What, then, should you weigh? We have no exact measure of ideal body weight because the "norm" is based on population statistics, cultural perceptions, and the influence of genetically and environmentally determined differences in metabolism. In short, there are no absolute rules, only working guidelines:

Throughout this chapter we use the term "metabolism," which we define as the body processes, including a whole host of chemical reactions that are necessary to maintain function and sustain life.

- Men: 106 pounds for the first five feet, then add six pounds for every inch thereafter
- Women: 100 pounds for the first five feet, then add five pounds for every inch thereafter

Normal Diet. Food supplies us with carbohydrates, fats, and proteins that in turn supply energy. Energy is measured in calories. Carbohydrates and proteins provide approximately four calories per gram, and fat provides almost nine calories per gram—twice as much. People also need essential nutrients (such as certain vitamins, minerals, amino acids, and fatty acids) and other substances, such as fiber, from a *variety* of foods. Oranges, for example, are rich in vitamin C, bananas supply potassium, and a half-cup serving of cantaloupe contributes half of the daily requirement for beta-carotene.

> *I just read that lab tests at Cornell University show that natural chemicals in apples slow the growth rate of human liver cancer cells. The researchers said that they're not sure why, but it may be the antioxidants in fruits and vegetables—and it's best to eat a daily diet that includes five servings of a wide variety of fruits and vegetables.*
>
> *Ha! 'An apple a day' really does keep the doctor away.*
>
> *Bonnie*

A normal, healthy diet contains the amounts of essential nutrients and calories you need to prevent either a nutritional deficiency or excess and provides the right balance of carbohydrate, fat, and protein. Many Americans, however, don't have good eating habits. According to the Healthy Eating Index of the U.S. Department of Agriculture's (USDA) Center for Nutrition Policy and Promotion, only about 17 percent of people eat the recommended number of servings of fruit, and only about 31 percent eat the recommended number of servings of vegetables. In fact, diet-related health conditions (heart disease, stroke, cancer, and diabetes) "cost society about $250 billion annually in medical costs and lost productivity. Thirty to forty percent of deaths due to cancer can be prevented if people will choose a healthful diet and perform physical activity."[1]

What is a healthful diet? The USDA currently recommends a daily caloric intake of 30 to 40 calories per kilogram of body weight and the following dietary balance:

- 40 to 50 percent carbohydrate
- no more than 30 percent fat (less than 10 percent of calories from saturated fat)
- 1 to 1.5 grams of protein for each kilogram (2.2 lbs.) of body weight

For more information about healthy diets, I recommend you consult the Food Guide Pyramid published by the USDA. It graphically illus-

Food Guide Pyramid

A Guide to Daily Food Choices

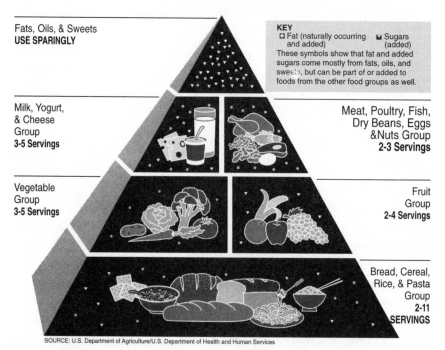

Fats, Oils, & Sweets
USE SPARINGLY

KEY
□ Fat (naturally occurring   ◹ Sugars
and added)   (added)
These symbols show that fat and added sugars come mostly from fats, oils, and sweets, but can be part of or added to foods from the other food groups as well.

Milk, Yogurt,
& Cheese
Group
3-5 Servings

Meat, Poultry, Fish,
Dry Beans, Eggs
&Nuts Group
2-3 Servings

Vegetable
Group
3-5 Servings

Fruit
Group
2-4 Servings

Bread, Cereal,
Rice, & Pasta
Group
**2-11
SERVINGS**

SOURCE: U.S. Department of Agriculture/U.S. Department of Health and Human Services

Use the Food Guide Pyramid to help you eat better every day. . . the Dietary Guidelines way. Start with plenty of Breads, Cereals, Rice, and Pasta; Vegetables; and Fruits. And two to three servings from the Milk group and two to three servings from the Meat

Each of these food groups provides some, but not all, of the nutrients you need. No one food group is more important than another — for good health you need them all. Go easy on fats, oils, and sweets, the foods in the small tip of the Pyramid.

To order a copy of "The Food Guide Pyramid" booklet, send a $1.00 check or money order made out to the Superintendent of Documents to: Consumer Information Center, Department 1599-Y, Pueblo, Colorado 81009.

U.S. Department of Agriculture, Human Nutrition Information Service, August 1992, Leaflet No. 572

trates the importance of balance among different food groups in a daily eating pattern and suggests the number (depending on daily calorie intake desired) and size of daily servings. As you can see, you should choose a variety of grains (especially whole grains), fruits, and vegetables.

Pyramid serving sizes are not large. For example, one serving equals one-half cup of pasta; one cup of raw, leafy vegetables; one-half cup of other vegetables (cooked or chopped raw); one medium apple, banana, orange; one cup of milk or yogurt; or two to three ounces of cooked lean meat, poultry, or fish.

The USDA recommendations include a range of servings from each of the five major food groups. People who consume about 1,600 calories a day should be guided by the smaller number; the larger number is for people who are very active and consume about 2,800 calories a day:

- Choose most of your daily foods from the bread, cereal, rice, and pasta group (6–11 servings), vegetable group (3–5 servings), and fruit group (2–4 servings).
- Choose moderate amounts of foods from the milk, yogurt, and cheese group (2–3 servings) and the meat, poultry, fish, dry beans, eggs, and nuts group (2–3 servings).
- Limit foods that provide few nutrients and are high in fat and sugar.
- In general, the USDA recommends a diet that is low in saturated fat and cholesterol and moderate in total fat. The new 2000 guidelines also urge you to choose appropriate beverages and foods in order to moderate your intake of sugars and salt.

Resource: For a free copy of *Dietary Guidelines for Americans,* call the USDA Center for Nutrition Policy and Promotion Publication Line: 202-606-8000 or write to 1120 20th St., NW, Suite 200, North Lobby, Washington, DC 20036. Website: www.usda.gov/cnpp

Resource: The American Dietetic Association's (ADA) National Referral Line (to find qualified dieticians in your area) is 1-800-366-1655. Helpful books: *Complete Food & Nutrition Guide* by Roberta Duyff and ADA and *Dieting for Dummies* by Jane Kirby and ADA. Website: www.eatright.org

Resource: The American Institute for Cancer Research provides practical tips on good nutrition with its newsletter, pamphlets (ask for "The New American Plate" brochure), and a toll-free AICR Nutrition Hotline staffed by a registered dietician: Call 1-800-843-8114 and request Nutrition Information. Website: www.aicr.org

Resource: *Nutrition Action Health Letter* (Center for Science in the Public Interest). Website: www.cspinet.org

Resource: Track your "5 a day" minimum number of fruits and vegetables for a healthy diet and the average number of minutes you spend on daily exercise, along with recipes and tips for a healthy lifestyle at a website run by the National Cancer Institute and the CDC. Website: www.5aday.nci.nih.gov

Nutrition and the Liver

The liver is the major organ responsible for regulating and responding to your body's metabolic demands. Your liver must be functioning well to maintain normal metabolism of carbohydrates, fats, and protein; it is also responsible for processing and using several vitamins. This section deals with the role a healthy liver (and a healthy, well-balanced diet) plays in these nutritional processes.

Carbohydrate Metabolism. The most common sources of dietary carbohydrate are sugars, such as sucrose (table sugar), fructose (corn syrup), and lactose (milk sugar), and starches, such as breads, pasta, grains, cereals, fruits, vegetables, and potatoes. When you eat carbohydrates, specialized enzymes in the pancreas and gut process them to yield simple sugars (glucose, galactose, fructose, maltose).

These sugars are absorbed by intestinal lining cells, enter the portal circulation, and travel to the liver via the portal vein. During overnight fasting, blood sugar levels dip to a relatively low level, insulin secretion is suppressed, and blood insulin levels diminish. After a meal, blood sugar increases (stimulating the release of insulin from the pancreas), and insulin levels rise. Insulin, which rises in response to a meal, is the hormone that stimulates the liver to take in more glucose and to move the glucose into storage—mainly in the form of glycogen. The liver can then release glycogen to your muscles for energy during periods of fasting or exercise.

Although the liver can store considerable amounts of glycogen, it is the first energy source used during periods of prolonged fasting or caloric deprivation, and it can be depleted rapidly. After glycogen, the body taps other energy sources—including protein and fat.

Protein Metabolism. We take in dietary protein from dairy products, produce, and meats. Enzymes produced by the pancreas and intestine break down the protein into its amino acids and small peptides. The intestine rapidly absorbs the amino acids with specific transport systems

TABLE 5A. SOME COMMON LIVER PROTEINS AND THEIR
FUNCTION IN THE HUMAN BODY

Protein	Function
Clotting Factors (II, V, VII, IX, and X)	Maintain normal clotting
Albumin	Maintain normal blood volume
Renin	Regulate blood pressure
Binding globulins	Regulate hormone action
Transferrin	Transport iron
Ferritin	Store iron
Retinol binding protein	Transport Vitamin A to the eye
LDL receptor	Remove Cholesterol from the blood
P-450 proteins	Metabolize drugs, chemicals, toxins

within its lining cells and then delivers the amino acids to the liver via the portal vein.

When they reach the liver, they are used for energy or for making (synthesizing) new proteins. The newly synthesized proteins perform specific body functions (see Table 5A).

Fat Metabolism. In general, fats are neutral lipids (triglycerides), acidic lipids (fatty acids), and sterols (cholesterol, plant sterols). Triglycerides (dairy products, meats, oils, butter, margarine) are the most common type of dietary fat and represent a major source of energy. The liver is uniquely suited to regulate and process triglycerides.

Dietary triglyceride is digested in the intestine by lipase, an enzyme secreted by the pancreas in response to meals. Bile, secreted by the liver, makes the digested fat soluble and promotes its absorption. Absorbed fat is then repackaged and transported into blood, where the liver ultimately removes it from the circulation. Fat that reaches the liver is processed in three ways: (1) stored as fat droplets in liver cells, (2) metabolized as a source of energy, and (3) repackaged, secreted back into blood, and delivered to other cells in the body.

The liver is also intimately involved with the processing of dietary cholesterol and is the main source of newly synthesized cholesterol in the body. Liver disease may be associated with both high or low blood cholesterol levels. In general, as liver disease progresses in patients with hepatitis B, the blood level of cholesterol drops.

Bile. The liver produces and secretes a fluid (bile) that enters the intestine to aid in digestion and absorption. Bile is clear yellow to golden-brown and contains water, electrolytes (salts), cholesterol, bile salts (detergents), phospholipids, and proteins. Bile helps to activate enzymes secreted by the pancreas and is essential for the digestion and absorption of fat or fat-soluble vitamins.

Vitamins. The liver plays a role in several steps of vitamin metabolism. I'll describe only a few of those steps. Vitamins are either fat-soluble (Vitamins A, D, E, and K) or water-soluble (Vitamin C and the B-complex vitamins).

Patients with advanced liver disease may become deficient in water-soluble vitamins, but this is usually due to inadequate nutrition and poor food intake. Vitamin B12 storage usually far exceeds the body's requirements; deficiencies rarely occur due to liver disease or liver failure. When dietary intake drops, however, thiamine and folate commonly become deficient. Oral supplementation is usually all that you need to restore thiamine and folate stores to the normal range.

Fat-soluble vitamins require not only adequate dietary intake but also good digestion and absorption by the body. That's why normal production of bile is essential. Bile in the gut is required for the absorption of fat-soluble vitamins into the body because these vitamins are relatively insoluble in water. Bile acts as a detergent, breaking down and dissolving these vitamins so they may be properly absorbed.

If bile production is poor, oral supplementation of Vitamins A, D, E, and K may not be sufficient to restore vitamin levels to normal. The use of a detergent-like solution of liquid Vitamin E (TPGS) improves the absorption of Vitamin E in patients with advanced liver disease. The same solution may also improve the absorption of Vitamins A, D, and K if the latter are taken simultaneously with the liquid Vitamin E.

Nutritional Needs for Hepatitis B Patients Who Don't Have Cirrhosis

Caloric Requirements. In general, the noncirrhotic patient with hepatitis B has caloric needs similar to those of noninfected people of the same age and gender. For this reason we recommend the following:

- no salt restriction
- no protein restriction

- 30 to 40 calories per kilogram intake per day
- one multivitamin per day

Patients who drink excessive amounts of alcohol should stop drinking altogether. They may also need supplementation with thiamine and folate.

Patients often proudly tell me that they are restricting their protein intake to "help" their livers. I'd like to emphasize that moderate amounts of protein (as recommended by the Food Pyramid) should be a normal part of your diet. If you are concerned about fat content, choose low-fat sources of protein. Protein restriction is recommended only for patients with cirrhosis who have encephalopathy (mental confusion).

Common questions I'm asked are, "Will dietary fat harm my liver? Should I avoid fat? Can I digest fat?" Dietary fat (triglycerides) undergoes complex processing (see Chapter 4). In the setting of liver disease, fat may accumulate in the liver. However, dietary fat intake does not correlate with the degree of fatty accumulation. Nonetheless, liver fat (steatosis) may promote liver injury and fibrosis in patients with viral hepatitis. Therefore, we do recommend a diet relatively low in fat, particularly saturated fat.

On the other hand, viral hepatitis by itself does not alter fat digestion or absorption from the gut. Only patients with advanced liver disease (cirrhosis) with jaundice have altered fat digestion and absorption. Jaundice in the setting of cirrhosis indicates severe impairment of processing and secretion of bile. Reduced bile concentration in the gut limits fat digestion and absorption.

Vitamin Supplements. In general, noncirrhotic patients with hepatitis B do not require any additional vitamin supplementation other than that noted above. One concern is that if bile production drops, the patient may become deficient in fat-soluble vitamins during the course of hepatitis B infection. This deficiency rarely develops during the early stages of hepatitis B, but it may be fairly prevalent at later, cirrhotic stages of the disease. When detected, deficiencies of fat-soluble vitamins should be corrected by administering proper doses of the compounds.

I am frequently asked, "Is it okay to take iron?" The answer goes beyond a simple yes or no. Women who are actively ovulating tend to lose iron through menstruation. Some of these women may develop iron deficiency and anemia, and they may actually benefit from iron.

Men and non-ovulatory or post-menopausal women typically are not iron-deficient, and supplementation is not necessary. In fact, inappropriate supplementation with iron-loaded vitamins may be harmful in patients with liver disease.

One theory of the development of liver disease is that oxidant stress promotes liver cell injury and also stimulates specialized cells in the liver (stellate cells) to produce the main fibrosis protein, collagen. Iron is a catalyst for oxidant injury by promoting formation of "free radicals" that can initiate injury and fibrosis.

Supplemental Vitamin C may be of potential benefit because it has anti-oxidant properties. However, Vitamin C may promote iron absorption and lead to excessive accumulation of iron in the liver. The latter effect could actually increase oxidant injury. A reasonable, middle-ground approach is to take in the daily FDA-recommended amount of Vitamin C and to avoid excessive supplementation.

Nutritional (Herbal) Therapies. According to the *Nutrition Business Journal*, supplements were a $15.4 billion dollar industry in 1999.[2] Patients with viral hepatitis have used a number of "nutritional supplements," such as echinaceae, pycnogenol, dandelion root, silymarin (milk thistle), and a wide array of herbal remedies. Most of these have not been studied in controlled trials and, thus, are unproved therapies. Silymarin has been studied but has not demonstrated clear benefit.

Despite the lack of supporting data, the use of these therapies has gained widespread acceptance among patients with viral hepatitis. Several factors seem to account for this phenomenon: a history of lack of effective therapies for liver disease in general; incompletely effective treatment for hepatitis B; a general attitude that, "It's 'natural' so it can't hurt me, and maybe it'll help;" and the relatively mild and slowly progressive nature of hepatitis B.

Herbs have been used to treat illness since time began. In fact, many modern pharmaceuticals were discovered in natural sources. Aspirin originally came from the bark of the white willow tree. Cyclosporin, the miracle drug that suppresses the immune system and makes liver transplants possible, was found in a fungus growing in the soil of a plateau in southern Norway.

I have no doubt that future controlled studies of herbs for liver disease will result in useful treatments. Saw palmetto, for example, has been studied in a controlled trial by New York University researchers and found effective in certain doses for prostate conditions. Some "natural" substances are ineffective, and others may be as powerful as approved Western medicines. However, until we have proof of effectiveness and safety, I cannot endorse or recommend that patients undergo nutritional therapies.

Quality control of potency and contaminants is another problem. In 1998, California investigators found that "nearly one-third of 260 imported Asian herbals were either spiked with drugs not listed on the label or contained lead, arsenic or mercury."[3]

In addition, herbs can interact with other medications you may be taking. For example, St. John's wort, a popular herbal antidepressant, recently has been found to decrease levels of life-sustaining cyclosporine in heart transplant patients.[4]

I do not recommend using herbs, but if you are interested in them, become informed. And remember that it is vitally important to tell your doctor if you are taking any nutritional supplement.

Under current laws, herbs classified as food or dietary supplements are exempt from regulations governing quality control and proof of effectiveness. Often, people will take the recommendations of the clerk who sells the supplements.

> I went to a health food store and asked them to give me anything that would help my liver. I bought coltsfoot, comfrey, petasites, chaparral, and yohimbe.
>
> My enzymes shot up to 800. When the doctor asked me if I was taking anything new, I brought in the bottles and learned that these herbs were best avoided because they may be toxic for the liver. I stopped taking them, and my enzymes went back down.
>
> Harold

Why isn't more research done on herbs? In 1978, the German government set up Commission E. The agency doesn't conduct research, but it does review studies and other evidence of safety and effectiveness, including anecdotal reports, and publishes its findings. Congress responded to the public interest and increased funding for the National Institutes of Health (NIH) Center for Complementary and Alternative Medicine/Office of Alternative Medicine from $50 million for fiscal year 1999 to $68.7 million for fiscal year 2000. The largest portion of the funding goes to herbal product research.

In 1994 Congress passed the Dietary Supplement Health and Education Act (DSHEA) that gave dietary supplement manufacturers the freedom to market more products. The Food and Drug Administration (FDA) must review clinical studies of drugs to determine effectiveness, safety, dosages, and possible interactions with other substances. Under DSHEA, however, the FDA does not authorize or test dietary supplements, and manufacturers do not need the agency's approval of ingredients and products before marketing.

Herbs Harmful to the Liver. After a dietary supplement is on the market, the FDA has the responsibility for showing that it is unsafe before it can take action to restrict use. In June 1997 the FDA proposed to limit the amount of ephedrine alkaloids in dietary supplements (marketed as ephedra, Ma Huang, Chinese ephedra, and epitonin, for example) and to provide warnings to consumers about hazards (including hepatitis) associated with use of these substances.[5]

In 1993 the FDA named before a Senate committee other supplements as possible hazards associated with illness and injuries to the liver. The list includes Chaparral, Comfrey, Germander, Vitamin A (in doses of 25,000 or more International Units a day), and Niacin (in slow-release doses of 500 mg. or more a day or immediate-release doses of 750 mg. or more a day).

Here is a list I give to my patients of herbs that have been documented to cause liver problems, ranging from hepatitis to liver failure: Atractylis Gummifera, Azadirachza indica, Berberis vulgaris, Callilepsis laureola, Cassia angustifolia (Senna), Crotalaria, Corydalis, Hedeoma pulegoides, Heliotropium, Larrea tridentata (Chaparral bush, Creosote bush, Greasewood), Lycopodium serratum (Jin Bu Huan), Mentha pulegoides, Sassafras albidum (Sassafras), Scuteileria (Skullcap), Stephania, Symphytum officinale (Comfrey), Teucrium chamaedrys [Germander (mint family)], Tussilago farfara (Peppermint), Valeriana officinalis (Valerian, Asfetida, Hops, Gentian), Viscum alba [Mistletoe, Margosa oil, Mate tea, Gordolobo yerba tea, Pennyroyal (squawmint) oil];[6] Senecio, Heliotropium, Chelidonum majus (greater celandine), and "a variety of Chinese herbal mixtures (artemisia, hare's ear, chrysanthemum, plantago seed, gardinia, red peony root, etc.").[7]

In my opinion, if you have a chronic liver disease, such as hepatitis B, you should avoid herbs that have not been tested in controlled studies, especially if you are being treated with interferon. Any substance, such as herbs or over-the-counter medications, may interact with drugs you are taking. Always discuss medicines and herbs with your physician.

Resource: Food and Drug Administration, Office of Consumer Affairs, HFE-88, Rockville, MD 20857. Consumer Food Information Line (Center for Food Safety and Applied Nutrition Outreach and Information Center): 1-800-FDA-4010 (in Washington, D.C., call 202-205-4314). FDA Website:
www.cfsan.fda.gov/~dms/supplmnt.html

Resource: National Institutes of Health (NIH) Center for Complementary and Alternative Medicine/Office of Alternative Medicine Clearinghouse 1-888-644-6226. Website:
http://altmed.od.nih.gov

Resource: The National Digestive Disease Information Clearinghouse (NDDIC) offers a brochure, "Harmful Effects of Medicines on the Adult Digestive System," which describes some over-the-counter and prescription drugs that may affect the liver. Call 301-654-3810. Website: www.niddk.nih.gov

Resource: Tyler, Varro E. *The Honest Herbal: A Sensible Guide to the Use of Herbs and Related Remedies.* New York: Pharmaceutical Products Press. 1993.

Resource: Gruenwald, Joerg, Thomas Brendler, Christof Jaenicke. *PDR® for Herbal Medicines.* Montvale: Medical Economics. 2000.

Nutrition Tips from Patients.
People with hepatitis who are interested in nutrition find many ways to work toward healthier eating habits. Here are some of their suggestions:

> *I started checking how much I eat by actually measuring a cup of cereal in the morning. Was I surprised. A cup is a lot smaller portion than I was used to eating, let me tell you. After a while, I got so I could eyeball sane-sized portions, and I didn't have to measure anymore.*

> *I never drink alcohol anymore. I just took it out of the picture. If you mix alcohol and hepatitis, you're asking for trouble.*

> *I don't eat raw oysters—or any raw fish or meat, for that matter. They can be contaminated with hepatitis A or the bacteria that causes cholera. Hepatitis A is really bad for people who already have hepatitis B.*

I think vitamins and minerals in REAL foods are the best way to go. But sometimes I get nauseous, and it's hard to eat. That's when I think a multivitamin without iron helps.

Fatty foods don't seem to digest well and cause gas. If I eat sugary foods, such as pancakes and syrup, I can bet on a drastic drop in energy in about two hours. My theory is that my damaged liver can't regulate the sugar in my blood too well so when I indulge my sweet tooth, it sends my body into sugar high and low extremes. I feel better eating low-fat protein foods, such as lean meat, beans, skim milk, etc. I start each day with a couple of spoonfuls of protein powder, and that seems to give me a smooth supply of energy into the afternoon hours.

It was really hard to give up coffee. First I switched to decaf. Now I'm into this ginger-honey syrup. I put a little bit into a cup of hot water. Sometimes I add lemon. My liver thanks me every day.

I used to take megadoses of vitamin C. Then I read that C helps your body absorb iron. I buy a daily multivitamin pill that doesn't have iron, because I don't want to overload my liver. Well, it doesn't make sense to take extra C then, does it?

When I eat out, I have what I call my "rule of half." Restaurant portions are too big so I try to eat only half. Well, I don't always make it, but I try.

One thing I feel "well" on is homemade soup. I make a big kettle of soup and keep it in the fridge for small meals. I boil beef, chicken, or turkey and skim off the fat. I put in canned tomatoes, peppers, bok choy, parsnips, zucchini, or any other vegetable I have around. Then I season it. Except for the potatoes, you get a low-carbohydrate, low-fat, moderate protein, nutritious brew that you can eat all day long if you want.

Eating small meals several times a day works better for me than eating a few large meals because sometimes I get nauseous, and I don't have much appetite.

I carry snack-size bags of dry cereal with me in case I get hungry. I used to be a candy-holic, and the cereal is a healthy substitute. My friend teases me, though. She says it's what she used to do for her kids when they were babies.

Drink LOTS of water. Period. Stay away from drinks with empty calories.

I always drank soda. It was nothing for me to down four or five cans of pop a day. But when I started checking labels, I couldn't believe it—salt, sugar, preservatives. It took me a while to pare down and switch to water, but I don't drink pop at all now.

I read a lot about diet and nutrition, and the other day I read that a large glass of purple grape juice a day offers most of the same heart protection as red wine. As a hepster, I don't drink alcohol so this was great news. It just occurred to me that I could simply eat more red and purple grapes, too.

Nutritional Needs for Hepatitis B Patients with Cirrhosis

Caloric Requirements. In general, the patient with early-stage or compensated cirrhosis still requires 30 to 40 calories per kilogram a day. You may need to alter your dietary habits to take in this number of calories, because as hepatitis B progresses to cirrhosis, you may begin to experience loss of appetite, increasing fatigue, reduction in physical activity, and alteration of your sleep-wake pattern. People commonly complain of loss of exercise tolerance ("I'm just too pooped out to get my work done"). In addition, these changes often precipitate a sense of despondency, anxiety, or depression. It helps to develop both a pattern of meals that allows you to use your diet for maximum energy and a rest pattern that reduces prolonged periods of physical activity.

No nutritional prescription is right for every patient. You need to address your specific nutritional needs with your physician. In my experience, patients with hepatitis B who develop compensated cirrhosis benefit by more frequent, smaller volume meals. Instead of one or two large meals, divide the equivalent amount of calories into four smaller meals. In addition, supplementation with one or two tablets of multivitamins is generally indicated, although the overall benefit is unclear. Despite this change in dietary habit, fatigue often persists. People benefit from "rest periods," usually 30 minutes or an hour in the mid-afternoon.

Caution: Please understand that advanced cirrhosis is associated with severe impairment of liver function and that specific dietary modifications may be necessary and could alter the general guidelines noted above. Your doctor may recommend a consultation with a dietician or provide you with a specific nutritional prescription.

Protein Restriction. It is important that the patient with cirrhosis take in enough protein to avoid excessive muscle wasting and energy depletion. However, if encephalopathy develops, a doctor might prescribe a "protein-restricted" diet.

Encephalopathy is the alteration or cloudiness of mental function. When the condition is severe, the patient becomes disoriented, confused, combative, or even comatose. Encephalopathy may also cause altered sleep-wake patterns, altered personality, and lack of motor coordination.

One factor contributing to these symptoms is dietary protein intake, so patients with any of the above symptoms may be placed on protein restrictions. This diet is usually not zero protein, but a reduced level of 20 to 60 grams per day. Often, the physician will use other treatments in conjunction with this diet, such as lactulose or neomycin.

It's not that protein is bad for me. It's that the liver is unable to process the protein that my body takes in. I think this shows up in real numbers—in my case, ammonia levels up to 12 times higher than the norm. That leads to less capacity for memory, balance, and general coping.

With those numbers I have more abdominal pain, ascites, depression, itching, muscle twitches, and hypersensitivity to odors that normally don't bother me.

Christopher

Vitamin Supplements. Most people with hepatitis B, even those with cirrhosis, have adequate intake and storage of water-soluble vitamins (C, B complex). To be sure, I recommend the addition of two tablets of multivitamins each day (one in the morning and one in the evening).

Patients who excessively use or abuse alcohol risk becoming deficient in these vitamins, particularly thiamine and folate, and they may benefit from taking supplements. As I have emphasized before, the hepatitis B patient should avoid alcohol. Those who avoid alcohol probably won't require either supplement.

Mineral Supplements. Patients with cirrhosis may experience deficiencies in three minerals: calcium, magnesium, and zinc. Calcium deficiency may be related to a lack of Vitamin D, poor nutrition, or malabsorption. Correcting the underlying abnormality may be all that is required to restore calcium balance. However, bone thinning may occur even without these specific problems, so I recommend 0.5 to 1.0 grams of calcium each day. Calcium may be taken in the form of dairy products or therapeutic supplements. When the patient can't take in enough dairy products because of protein, salt, or fluid restrictions (see next section), supplements are used.

Magnesium deficiency may occur due to inadequate dietary intake. However, it occurs more often when patients take diuretics to treat fluid retention because their kidneys flush out the magnesium as waste. Symptoms of magnesium deficiency include muscle cramps, fatigue, weakness, nausea, and vomiting. Often, it's not possible to modify or discontinue diuretics in cirrhotic patients, so magnesium supplementation (500 mg. magnesium gluconate three times a day) may be required.

Zinc deficiency may cause the loss of the senses of smell and taste. Patients with these symptoms may benefit from supplementation with zinc sulfate (220 mg. three times a day).

Salt and Fluid Restriction. Cirrhosis disturbs the regulation of body salt and water. Severe liver disease generates neural and hormonal signals to the kidney that cause the kidney to retain both salt and water. The salt acts like a sponge. As a result, fluid accumulates in certain tissues and body spaces, such as the ankles (peripheral edema), abdomen (ascites), and chest (pleural effusion).

I preach from a salt-box! Six months after I was diagnosed with hepatitis B, my legs were swollen, and my belly was tight as a drum. By limiting my salt intake to 500 mg. a day (with occasional days for "cheating") my ascites has been kept at bay, and I only have to take minimal medications for it.

TABLE 5B. 2-GRAM SALT DIET SAMPLE MENU*

Breakfast (352–765 mg)
    1–2 pieces toast (150–400 mg)
    1–2 tsp. margarine (50 mg)
    1 Tbs. orange marmalade
    1 boiled egg (62 mg)
        or 1 fried egg (162 mg)
    1 C cooked cereal with little or no salt (1 mg)
    ½–1 C milk (60–120 mg)
    6 oz. brewed coffee (4 mg)/tea (5 mg)/herbal tea (2 mg)
    1 C cantaloupe (14 mg) or strawberries (2 mg)
    1 C orange juice (2 mg)

Lunch (503–611 mg)
    3.5 oz. salmon patty (96 mg)
    1 slice tomato (½ mg) and ½ C lettuce (1 mg)
    1 oz. potato chips (about 10 chips) (170 mg)
    1 C fresh grapes (2 mg)
    1 C apple juice (7 mg)
    1 carrot (25 mg) and 1 stalk of celery (35 mg)
    1 piece angel food cake [161 mg (homemade); approx. 270 mg (packaged mix)]
    8 oz. ice tea (5 mg) with lemon (less than 1 mg)

Dinner (431–601 mg)
    3.5 oz. roast beef (63–73 mg) au jus with no added salt (if packaged
        gravy mix, 2 oz. = approx. 160 mg)
    1 baked potato (16 mg)
    1 Tbsp. sour cream (6 mg)/margarine (100 mg)
    ½ C frozen green beans (3 mg)
    1½ C tossed fresh salad (5 mg) with salt-free salad dressing
    1 piece apple pie (181 mg) with ½ C vanilla ice cream (53 mg)
    6 oz. coffee (4 mg)

*Sodium levels generally refer to fresh homemade items, are approximate, and vary with brand names of products used. Fast, pre-packaged, or canned foods usually contain much higher levels of sodium.

Most people have a heavy hand with salt. A pancake breakfast at a restaurant has more sodium than I allow myself for the whole day. But I can make pancakes at home using salt-free butter and going light on the milk and eggs for one-third of my daily salt allotment.

Jonathon

Treatment of fluid retention always requires dietary salt restriction, often requires diuretics (medicines that block the kidney and cause increased urination of salt and water), and sometimes requires fluid restriction. Patients need to understand that the major driving force behind the accumulation of fluid is the excessive retention of salt. Diuretics work because they cause the kidney to lose salt. If you take in too much salt in your diet, you'll cause more fluid to accumulate in your body. In other words, you can override the effects of the diuretics, and patients on diuretics can actually retain fluid if they don't comply with a salt-restricted diet.

The usual salt restriction is two grams per day (see Table 5B). Commonly used diuretics are Aldactone® (spironolactone), Midamor® (amiloride), Lasix® (furosemide), HCTZ® (hydrochlorothiazide), and Zaroxylyn® (metolozone). Aldactone® and Midamor® conserve potassium, while Lasix®, HCTZ®, and Zaroxylyn® waste potassium. Most of the time, a doctor will prescribe the two types of diuretics together to minimize any changes in blood potassium levels. Occasionally, potassium supplements are used to keep blood potassium in the normal range.

The physician usually orders fluid restriction only for edematous patients with low levels of sodium in their blood. Fluid restriction means restriction of all fluids: water, tea, coffee, milk, etc. Patients with severe symptomatic low blood sodium may find it necessary to restrict their fluid intake to less than one quart a day.

Caution: Always consult with your physician regarding use of diuretics (doses and frequency) or dietary restrictions on salt or fluid intake. It is potentially dangerous to self-medicate or introduce dietary restrictions without physician consultation.

He who keeps on eating after his stomach is full digs his grave with his teeth.

Turkish proverb

References

[1] "Q and A's on Dietary Guidelines for Americans, 2000." 3 June 2000, *Center for Nutrition Policy and Promotion.* 1 Sept. 2000 www.usda.gov/cnpp/Pubs/DG2000/Qa5-2.pdf

[2] "NBJ's Fifth Annual Overview of the Nutrition Industry," *Nutrition Business Journal* Vol. V No.7/8 2000:1.

[3] Guy Gugliotta, "Supplements Aren't So Healthy," *Denver Post* March 19, 2000: 5A.

[4] T.H. Breidenbach, M.W. Hoffman, T.H. Becker, H. Schlitt, J. Klempnauer. "Drug Interaction of St. John's Wort with Cyclosporine." *Lancet.* 27 May 2000; 355:1912.

[5] Paula Kurtzweil, "An FDA Guide to Dietary Supplements," *FDA Consumer* Sept.-Oct. 1998:29.

[6] D. Larrey, G. P. Pageaux. "Hepatotoxicity of Herbal Remedies and Mushrooms." Seminars in Liver Disease. 1995; 15:183-188.

[7] D. Schuppan, J.D. Jia, B. Brinkhaus, E.G. Hahn. "Herbal Products for Liver Diseases: A Therapeutic Challenge for the New Millennium." *Hepatology.* 1999; 30:1100.

6

TAKING CARE OF YOURSELF EMOTIONALLY

Emotional Challenges of Chronic Illness

I've been through a hellava lot. I was diagnosed with a life-threatening disease. I completely freaked out when I found that I inadvertently infected my daughter with hepatitis B. Thank God she recovered! My marriage ended. The fatigue and nausea got so bad, I had to quit my job.

I feel useless, and I don't want to be a drag on my family. How does a person cope? How do you live with this disease so that you don't become the disease?

Terry

I N   T H I S   C H A P T E R , we draw on the expertise of mental health professionals who work with hepatitis patients. We also present the experiences of the patients themselves. Who else really understands? Here are the topics we'll cover:

- Phase 1: Diagnosis
- Special Problems with a Diagnosis of Hepatitis B
- Phase 2: Impact (Attitudes and Expectations)

- Phase 3: Reorganization
- Healing vs. Curing
- Warning Signs of Depression
- Understanding your Family and Friends (Family Systems)
  Boundaries
- Tools for Wellness: Some Practical Suggestions
  Medical Care and Psychological Help
  Support Groups
  Exercise and Nutrition
  Feeling Useful/Having Fun
  Exploring Your Creative and Spiritual Sides

Hepatitis B may be the biggest emotional challenge you'll ever face. How do you deal with chronic disease without letting it take over your life?

"The goal is balance," says Meredith Pate-Willig, a licensed clinical social worker. Ms. Pate-Willig facilitates support groups for Denver's Qualife, an organization that seeks to enrich the quality of life for people facing life-challenging illness.

How do you achieve balance and a "wellness lifestyle?" "There's no short cut through normal, natural cycles of grief," says Pate-Willig. "Grieving is nature's way of helping us adapt to new information about our illness."

Too often, we're hard on ourselves as we grieve. In a world of instant cereal and microwave popcorn, we think we should be grieving faster, better. The truth is, each one of us goes through the process in our own time frame and in our own way—and the healing ingredient is kindness. Be patient with yourself. You will work it through, and you will come out of the crisis with a stronger sense of who you are.

According to Pate-Willig, it's helpful to think of these spiraling cycles of grief in three phases: diagnosis, impact, and reorganization.

Phase 1: Diagnosis

Diagnosis plunges you into a state of disbelief or shock.

> *I made an appointment with a specialist only to satisfy my family doctor. When he told me I was sick, my first thought was, "I'm so healthy!" I was in denial. I just didn't believe him. My husband was in shock.*
>
> *Martha*

If you lose your image of yourself as a healthy person, and you struggle or rebel against becoming a patient, how do you adjust? Some patients develop a sense of grief. Grieving is one way we work through loss, whether it's loss of our old selves ("I used to cook big family dinners. Now I'm too tired.") or loss of our dreams ("Will I ever marry now? Know my grandchildren? Launch a new business?"). According to Pate-Willig, "Grieving is normal—even necessary. It's the bridge between what was to what is. If you don't go across that bridge, you may face a continuing struggle."

In this first phase of diagnosis, you need your family and support system to pull together to help you adjust:

1. The diagnosis may make you feel uncomfortable or leave you with a numbing sense of shock and loss. You should understand that this response is normal.
2. Everyone needs psychological and social support—not just the person with hepatitis B. Other family members may be affected by the diagnosis. When one part of a system changes, everything in the system reacts in a "ripple" effect.

People may not respond to you in the way that you anticipate or expect. You may process the information fast while family members take longer, or the reverse. How fast or how slowly people absorb the news affects the dynamics in a marriage or friendship—leaving everyone with the unconscious feeling that somehow the rules changed. In fact, just identifying these changes takes a while.

Sometimes, the patient or support system refuses to accept the new reality. "Denial," says Pate-Willig, "is a misunderstood defense. When it acts as a circuit-breaker, it keeps your system from overloading. That can be healthy. Denial becomes unhealthy when it keeps you from finding appropriate medical treatment."

Special Problems with a Diagnosis of Hepatitis B

Dealing with a diagnosis of any chronic illness is difficult, but patients with hepatitis B have special issues:

Feeling Low. You may be experiencing fatigue, low energy, loss of ability to concentrate, and a sense of inadequacy in doing daily tasks. These symptoms may make you more emotionally vulnerable and susceptible to periods of depression. Be sure to tell your doctor if you feel seriously depressed.

> *Today I woke up, made breakfast, and went back to bed. I had all these plans, but I'll do them tomorrow, not today. I've always been an active, intense person, and this is a big adjustment for me.*
>
> *Finally, though, I've got a name for this fatigue—a name I can give people. I tell them, "I've got hepatitis B, and I can't do that today. It wears me out quickly." In that way, it's a relief.*
>
> *Juan*

Feeling Contaminated. This is a difficult and sensitive topic. You may have questions and fears about infecting others. How will your friends or boss react? What do you tell your dentist?

> *I've learned not to share that I have hepatitis B because some people take it negatively. Honestly, I think I would too if I were on the other side.*
>
> *I've gone through phases. It's like death or divorce—the grieving, anger, and depression. It's like life. You just move on. I work. I have two kids. Maybe I appreciate life more.*
>
> *Sometimes I feel like I'm living with secrets. Hepatitis B is a part of me I don't share.*

> *I was diagnosed with hepatitis B about a week before my 25th wedding anniversary. The doctor told my husband that I had a sexually transmitted disease and that he should be tested and vaccinated. What the doctor failed to say was that this hepatitis could be spread in many other ways.*
>
> *I had complete trust in my husband. And thank God, he had faith and trust in me so the doctor suggesting I was sexually promiscuous did not harm our marriage.*

> *I was offered a job interpreting for a deaf child. I told the mother I had hepatitis B, and she wouldn't allow her daughter to be around me. I was turned down for quite a few jobs until one student said she was vaccinated, and it was no problem. We became friends over the years, and I'm going to her wedding in a few months.*

I'm a minister, and I live a very conservative lifestyle. I'm monogamous. I don't do drugs. I stood in front of my church, and said, "I have hepatitis B, and I want you all to be tested." After five years, I don't carry the guilt around anymore, because I warned everybody.

How You Got Infected. When you try to figure out how this happened to you, your answer may affect how you deal with your diagnosis: (1) If you can point to a blood transfusion, you don't feel responsible for your illness; (2) if you ever injected drugs, whether it was a minor episode or you're still involved, you have to process the painful idea that you did this to yourself; (3) if you were infected by a sexual partner, you may feel full of anger and distrust; (4) people who don't know how they got infected may never figure it out, and that uncertainty creates its own dilemmas.

I've tried for years to find out how I got the virus. Could it have been from my mother who died of liver cancer? Did I get it from dental work or surgeries or in one of the hospitals where I worked? Did I get it from the child who bit me while I was working in the schools?

I'll never know. The only thing I can be sure of is that I did not get hepatitis B from sexual contact, drug use, or tattoos. However, I've arrived at a place of peace in my life. I accept the fact that I'll never know—and I no longer search for that answer. Now I focus on how the virus can be stopped from spreading.

Betti

Looking Good. Strange as it sounds, people often have trouble offering comfort to someone who doesn't have a visible wound. In the early and middle stages of infection, you may suffer silent symptoms, such as fatigue and joint pains. Unfortunately, many people (including yourself) may have a hard time believing you're ill. Unless you explain the nature of hepatitis B, you may not get the support you need.

Fluctuating Nature of Hepatitis B. Who knows why a patient's hepatitis B DNA assay shows a low viral load one month but a sky-high level the next? The fluctuating course of hepatitis B sometimes gives the patient the feeling of walking on shifting sand, never knowing what each day will bring.

Lack of Information. Uncertainty due to lack of information is a huge stressor. You have no way to answer the questions, "What am I dealing with, and how will it affect my life?" What facts your doctor offers you about your stage of illness, therefore, have a big influence on how you deal with the diagnosis.

> *My wife died in September. In the spring my daughter and I took her ashes to California—to the ocean. We spread the ashes over the beach where she was so fond of walking. We did that in April, and when I got back, I had an annual physical.*
>
> *My liver enzymes were high, and a biopsy showed cirrhosis from hepatitis B. I could have gotten infected when I served in Korea or from blood transfusions after a horrendous auto accident more than 20 years ago. The virus took a long time to show itself.*
>
> *I've often wondered if my grief and despair at losing my wife didn't cause a defect in my immune system that allowed the virus, which was already there, to get worse and spread. Of course, I won't ever be able to prove it.*
>
> *Wayne*

What can you do to help yourself? "Be patient with yourself," says Pate-Willig. "Accept that this is a difficult time, and try not to beat yourself up for being normal, human.

"Remember to be kind to yourself. Patience, patience, and more patience. That's the key," says Pate-Willig. "Expect to feel emotional cycles, ups and downs, each time the activity of your disease changes or you experience a new symptom."

Phase 2: Impact (Attitudes and Expectations)

In Phase 1, the task for you and your support system is to pull together to confront and understand the new diagnosis. In the second phase, the question becomes, "How do we function now that we know that hepatitis B is a chronic condition? How do we gear up for the long haul?" It's a time of changing attitudes and expectations as you explore your options.

> *Seeing my boyfriend cope with hepatitis B made changes in me. He can't do some of the things he could do before. He was a late night person, but in the past year it's 8 p.m., and he's asleep.*

What's wrong with this picture? I had to adjust to his energy level.

It's rough for a single person. No one is lying next to you for you to say, "This is pretty rough for me," or to be held. You have to nurture yourself.

The challenge is how to connect with friends and family and still maintain the autonomy and space you need. Your questions may vary from large ("I'm a single parent with no one to care for me. Should I go back to my mom and dad's house or keep my own apartment?") to small ("My husband had a transplant. Should I play in my Thursday night bowling league or stay home with him?").

Families often have unspoken rules and myths about illness. Perhaps the message you got was, "Keep a stiff upper lip and don't show you're scared." Or maybe you grew up in a home where a cold meant deluxe pampering. What happens if you break these rules?

I'm a chronic carrier. When I told my husband I had hepatitis B, he turned to someone else who didn't have all the problems I have. He can't understand how much I worry about my children. What if something happens to me?

I talked about it too much, and he got angry. He resented me for hanging this over him. So now I don't talk about it with him anymore.

I owe a big debt to my companion. He never thought twice about my hepatitis B, about whether he would accept me into his life and home. He got vaccinated, and he's been very supportive.

Having somebody there to support me has been a big issue in my recovery. Those of us with hepatitis B owe a big thank you to our "hepper helpers," our spouses or partners.

Phase 3: Reorganization

As you move into Phase 3, you and your family begin to reorganize around the new reality. A sense of acceptance emerges, and you start to answer these questions: Who am I now? How am I going to make my life work?

At some point, things settle down. Perhaps you come to terms with a reduced energy level, make dietary changes, decide on a treatment plan.

Anything that tips the precarious balancing act shakes the system. If you start interferon treatment, you and your family and friends may need to organize around the treatment. Suppose you decide to plan a nap each day, while someone else assumes your chores. What most people don't realize is that any change, positive or negative, alters the system. So, paradoxically, you may need to reorganize after you have finished interferon treatment. For example, you may still feel the need for a daily nap, but the people around you may now disapprove.

The cycle of confronting the diagnosis, feeling its impact, and reorganizing yourself to deal with hepatitis B may recur with each piece of health news. If hepatitis B moves into advanced liver disease and a possible transplant, the concept of death may come to the forefront.

I'm Cherokee, and I have a Native American heritage from both my grandparents. My great-grandad was on the Trail of Tears.

When the hepatitis gets real bad, I sing my death song. It just comes to me. That relieves my pain, but I can't do it here in the hospital because they'd lock me up in a mental ward.

William

"The first big breakthrough for most people is the realization of how physically fragile we humans are," says Pate-Willig. "It's a difficult task to process, reprioritize, accept your mortality, and—at the same time—plan for post-transplant living."

Healing vs. Curing

"We are all desperate for curing," says Pate-Willig, "but a physical cure may be years away. We need to shift to healing—a balance and wholeness of mind, body, and spirit.

"As we become more aware of our emotional responses, we learn how healthy it is to lean into the grief process and accept it. We learn how to tap into resources, such as dietary changes and relaxation techniques. The goal is to come out of each cycle at a higher level, to feel better about ourselves, and to see more flexibility in ourselves and others as we learn how to cope."

Grief can be the great healer. Grief is to the psyche and the spirit what the physical process is to the healing of a wound.

So, you say, "That sounds great. But how do I grieve?"

"Talk about what's happening to you," says Pate-Willig. Talk to a friend, a support group, a journal. Get on the Internet. Help yourself by re-evaluating your feelings each time you tell and retell your story. As you do this, you fit your new self into your old idea of yourself.

"The Chinese symbol for crisis is both danger and opportunity. Chronic illness can give us the opportunity to become deeper, broader, more flexible, and to find meaning in our lives."

Warning Signs of Depression

While grieving and depression are normal, sustained depression is not. Fortunately, there are many ways to treat depression with medications and "talk" therapy, so it's important to tell your doctor, advises Robert House, M.D., Director of Residency Training and the Department of Psychiatric Consultation Liaison Service for the University of Colorado Health Sciences Center.

What are the signs of depression? According to Dr. House, be on the alert for some of these symptoms, if they are changes from your normal behavior pattern:

- low energy, fatigue, lack of interest in your usual activities
- withdrawn and/or irritable behavior
- sleep disturbances that show a change in your routine pattern (such as sleeping less or more, waking up a lot, or waking earlier or later than usual, not rested and ready to begin the day)
- significant weight loss over a short period of time
- loss of appetite, food doesn't taste good
- tearfulness, breaking into tears for no apparent reason, "out of the blue"
- forming and talking about ideas of suicide, or a sense that life is not worth living
- feeling of hopelessness, helplessness that things won't get better
- reluctance to resume activities of daily living after a transplant (such as not getting along with your family, if you've always done so before; not resuming sexual relations with your spouse after a reasonable length of time; not dating, if single; isolating yourself from others)

Understanding Your Family and Friends (Family Systems)

Chronic illness is a family illness. When one member of a family becomes sick, it affects everyone. Normally, a family stays in balance with its own set of unwritten roles and rules. Roles involve position (Who is the breadwinner? Who takes out the garbage?). Roles always change as the patient needs to do less and shifts tasks to others. Rules are values; they can be about communication (Who can say what to whom?), emotion (Who is allowed to be sad?), education, sex, religion, and parenting.

Most important for people with hepatitis B are the family rules and values about health and illness. Problems arise when your family rules (or the rules of the family you grew up in) clash. How do you handle the medical system? Can you take time off if you have a cold or only if you're deathly ill?

> *When I'm talking with my husband, I say to myself, "At least I have this time." Life takes on a different kind of value. I cherish our talks; they are deep ones. He asks me, "How will things go? Will I be able to continue to work, to keep up my business?"*
>
> *He's a worker. He always worked long hours, but when his life changed, he said, "I really got the message that I bought what the outside world was saying—push, push, push yourself."*
>
> *He had to go inside and find a power greater than all of us. And you know what? He made the same amount of money the month he worked at home as he did the month before, even though he rested more and worked less!*
>
> *Kari*

Boundaries. Families create different boundaries. Some are so enmeshed that it's hard to tell where one member begins and another ends. They know how to pull together but need to learn how to allow outsiders to help. At the other end of the spectrum is the disengaged family where members have a high degree of autonomy and very little strong communication with each other. They need to learn how to draw closer together, so they can hear each other and support one another. Most families, of course, fall somewhere in between these two extremes. Chronic illness can cause disorganization, but this crisis can open more options and choices as the family modifies and changes its rules and values.

Families also go through life stages that have their own issues of separateness and connectedness, from the birth of a child to taking care of elderly parents. When illness occurs, it can disrupt the normal tasks of these life stages. Suppose, for example, that hepatitis B strikes a parent of a teenager. The teenager will feel pulled by conflicting forces: the need to separate and develop a life with peers versus the need to pull closer to the family. In this setting the adolescent must cope with developing separateness and freedom and providing more help with household or other chores.

Communication and openness are the keys to improving the level of understanding within your family. When family members talk about a problem in terms of shifts in roles, rules, and life stages, it diffuses the personal element. Usually, people feel hurt when a conflict arises because they think the other family members don't care about them. When you define the problem as a conflict in family roles, values, or degree of separation/connection, you can work toward a resolution.

Suppose, for example, that George wants his wife, Susan, to come with him to all his medical appointments. Meanwhile, Susan has had to take a part-time job to help pay the bills. Even though it's no one's fault, she's angry. Susan can't do it all, and her former role as the family's primary emotional support needs to be modified. Instead of blaming each other and feeling unloved, Susan and George talk about the role changes and come up with a compromise. Susan will go to the important medical appointments, and George will ask his sister to accompany him to the routine ones.

Do people want to change a family system? No, but illness brings unavoidable changes and, therefore, a feeling of loss of control. You can choose to be angry, or you can decide what can be changed and what cannot. How can we figure out a new system that's fair to everybody? What roles and values can we let go or modify?

Tools for Wellness: Some Practical Suggestions

Life-challenging illnesses, like hepatitis B, present opportunities for rethinking priorities. We may not always be able to cure the disease, but we can improve the quality of our lives. We can nourish ourselves by getting good medical and psychological care, exercising, eating nutritional foods, trying to live meaningful and useful lives, deepening relationships, having fun, and exploring our creative and spiritual sides.

As you explore, trust yourself to make choices that fit you. Hold on to your sense of balance and moderation. Some self-help philosophies may leave you feeling that somehow you failed if you can't "will away" or control the disease. Look for more realistic, gentler perspectives.

Adapt an open and curious attitude when exploring new areas, and don't try all of them at once. Make changes gradually. Here are some suggestions from Pate-Willig and others:

Caution: Specific recommendations regarding diet, nutrition, and exercise may vary and should be evaluated and discussed with your physician.

Medical and Psychological Help. Put together your medical team with care. The treatment of hepatitis B is evolving and requires knowledge of specialized tests and treatments. Many doctors don't have much experience with hepatitis B, so find a gastroenterologist or hepatologist who does. Most medical centers have doctors who specialize in liver disease (hepatologists) or can recommend appropriate community specialists.

Although credentials are important, effective therapy may also be dependent upon the doctor-patient relationship. Make sure that the two of you are a good fit. This is a very individual matter. Do you like your doctor to tell you exactly what to do, or do you prefer to have more input in decision making? Does the doctor answer your questions fully, or seem anxious to exit? Do the nurses and receptionist seem friendly and supportive?

> *I liked the first doctor I saw. He was highly qualified, but I had a bad feeling in my gut about the way the nurses hustled me in and out of the office. It was always quick-quick and hurry-hurry. And I began to worry that medical decisions would be made that way, too.*
>
> *After a lot of soul-searching, I switched to another doctor, a hepatologist. I got excellent care—the best—and the bonus was that the nurses were more in synch with my needs because they saw lots of patients with liver disease. I was nervous about giving myself interferon shots, and they were willing to spend a lot of time with me going over and over the instructions until I felt confident.*
>
> *I knew what I needed to get through interferon therapy—great medical care and a lot of support. And I made sure I got both.*
>
> *Celia*

If you need to see a mental health professional (psychologist, psychiatrist, social worker, professional counselor), get names from friends you trust and interview a few practitioners. Ask about their backgrounds and qualifications. Make sure they have experience in dealing with issues of chronic illness. They should be graduates of an accredited master's or Ph.D. program and licensed by the state as an independent practitioner or supervised by someone who is licensed.

Keep abreast of developments in hepatitis B research. The more you know, the better your decisions will be. (See Resources at the back of this book.) And finally, look at your own beliefs and attitudes about illness. Otherwise, you can't decide what works for you and what doesn't. We don't choose to be sick, but we can choose how we try to handle the situation.

Resources:

Bridges, William. *Transitions.* Reading: Addison-Wesley, 1980.

Clarke, Peter & Susan H. Evans. *Surviving Modern Medicine, How to Get the Best from Doctors, Family & Friends.* New Brunswick: Rutgers University Press, 1998.

Flach, Frederic, M.D. *Resilience: The Power to Bounce Back When the Going Gets Tough.* New York: Hatherleigh Press, 1997.

Kushner, Harold S. *When Bad Things Happen to Good People.* New York: Avon, 1981.

Travis, John W., M.D. and Regina Sara Ryan. *Wellness Workbook.* Berkeley: Ten Speed Press, 1988.

Support Groups. Many studies prove the importance of support systems. The results of one well-known study reported in 1989 by psychiatrist David Spiegel and colleagues showed that women with metastatic breast cancer who attended weekly group therapy sessions lived significantly longer than those who did not.[1]

Most of us benefit from a network of informal supportive relationships. Effective support always includes a sharing of emotions and feelings—a quality of reciprocity. Each person feels heard, validated, and has a sense of being able to draw upon that support, if necessary.

Formal support groups are useful because they provide a common experience for hepatitis B patients, information-sharing, a sense of not being alone, and a safe place to share feelings. Sometimes, however, it's difficult to attract enough members to make a hepatitis B group viable. Therefore, many people find an Internet e-mail list-serv or moderated chat room a helpful alternative. Use common sense. If the experience feels good, it's working for you. If you find yourself more upset and in a toxic situation, look for another group that meets your needs.

When I was first diagnosed, I joined a hepatitis support group. Pretty much everybody had hepatitis C; only one or two of us had B. At first it was helpful just to talk because we have some issues in common.

But B is different. The tests are more complicated to understand. It's more infectious, and it's definitely transmitted sexually. On the other hand, people with hepatitis C don't have a vaccine to protect their sexual partners and families.

Pretty soon the hep C people took over the group. After a while, I stopped going.

Helping others in my computer support group is a godsend. It keeps me busy. I could be a student forever, eternally. I love to use my mind. And I feel like I'm still able to do the nursing work I had to quit when I got sick.

I've gone through a lot of emotional and financial strain. If what I can share spares one person what I've had to experience, it's worth it!

Resource: Many organizations will refer you to support groups or help you start your own (see Resources at the back of this book). Call them or visit their Websites for information and help.

For people who don't live near a support group meeting, are housebound, or prefer the anonymity of a "virtual community," phone and online options are available:

Resource: The Hepatitis B Foundation lists the Hepatitis B Information and Support List in its newsletter, *B-Informed:*
http://www.geocities.com/Heartland/Estates/9350/hblist.html
To subscribe, send a blank email to: hepatitis-b-on@mail-list.com

(For online support groups for parents of children with hepatitis B, see Chapter 12.)

Resource: Contact Hepatitis Foundation International for a phone network called PATS (Patient Advocacy/Information). Phone: 1-800-891-0707 Email: HFI@intac.com Website: www.hepfi.org

Resource: The Hepatitis Neighborhood offers a Support Group Search of almost 500 groups listed by state and a weekly Town Hall chat room (on specific topics) supervised by nurses. Website: www.hepatitisneighborhood.com

Exercise and Nutrition. Physical movement not only strengthens your body, it helps your emotional state. If you can afford it, a personal trainer with experience in chronic illness is helpful. Hospitals often have cardiac or stroke rehabilitation experts who may be able to refer you to the right professional, but you don't need money to exercise. You can walk with a friend, rent a yoga or Tai Chi video, or try water exercise to avoid stress on painful joints. Be creative.

> *I exercise. I swim vigorously for an hour every morning—and I'm in my 70s. I walk, hike, and I spend my leisure time doing computer programming. It keeps my mind active.*
>
> *Jack*

For information on nutrition, see Chapter 5, Taking Care of Yourself Nutritionally.

Caution: Consult your doctor before you begin any exercise program or make dietary changes.

Feeling Useful/Having Fun. We need a sense of meaning and purpose in our lives. We also need to have fun and play. Look for activities that create joy, hope, and a sense of living fully. Balance is the key.

Ask yourself these questions: What is important to me? How am I acting on the important things in my life? How can I continue to have a meaningful existence within the limits of my health and energy levels?

> *I went from chronic persistent hepatitis B to chronic active, from fibrosis to cirrhosis. One doctor told me my liver would last for three years—and probably not that long. This was back in 1991, when they didn't do transplants for hepatitis B because it was so aggressive a disease. The only alternative was to accept death.*
>
> *I decided that whether I had six days, six years, or six months, I was going to get my master's degree. I wanted to make more of a contribution and also do something that would give my life meaning. I reread Victor Frankl's* Man's Search for Meaning. *He says it's not so much what's happening to us as the meaning we give to it.*
>
> *I went to school at night—slowly. It took me three years to get my counseling degree. I had fatigue, itching, nausea, bloating, muscle aches— but I got my adrenaline from working with patients. I helped start a hepatitis B support group, and I worked with AIDS patients. I saw people far worse off than I was.*

In 1995, I went on the transplant list. Then I read about lamivudine. It was being studied, and I begged my doctor to get it for me on a compassionate use basis. Within 30 days, my viral count went down to one percent. And now it's less than that. It took a couple of months, but I started to feel better.

George

Resources:

Anderson, Greg. *50 Essential Things to Do When the Doctor Says It's Cancer.* New York: Penguin, 1993.

LeShan, Lawrence. *Cancer As a Turning Point.* New York: Penguin, 1994.

Topf, Linda Noble with Hal Z. Bennett. *You Are Not Your Illness.* New York: Fireside, 1995.

Playing helps you recapture joy. "Like humor, a good joyful experience does as much for your sense of well-being as a good physical workout," says Pate-Willig. It requires flexibility and a commitment to explore options. If you can't climb mountains anymore, investigate handicapped-accessible trails or rent travel videos. Open yourself to new experiences. If you've never explored poetry, for example, now may be the time to visit your neighborhood library.

"Learn to live mindfully," says Pate-Willig. "Ask yourself: 'Do I notice the people chattering at my dinner table, and am I grateful for my family? Do I savor the vivid colors of the vegetables I'm cutting? Do I stop for a moment during the day to notice that I feel good?'"

Exploring Your Creative and Spiritual Sides. Using the mind's capacity for healing includes visualization, relaxation, guided imagery, meditation, journal writing, and creative arts. All of these are ways to help the mind create a quieter atmosphere and to improve your quality of life.

Alan did writing and journaling. He was meticulous about making entries. One day we looked at his book together, and in it he wrote how he was in a life and death struggle—and he chose life.

Sara

For me, Asian medicine seems compassionate. I take all my Western meds, but I also do self-massage on my liver and spleen. I take acupuncture, meditate, drink a special tea, and do healing movements much like Tai Chi. My sleeping disorder went away. I'm less bloated, and my skin is clear and bright.

Ed

Visualization, meditation, and relaxation create a sense of relaxed alertness and counteract the stress of daily living. Visit a bookstore and look over the tapes and videos. There are more than 30 methods, so the important thing is to find what makes you feel comfortable.

Resources:

Benson, Herbert and Miriam Klipper. *The Relaxation Response.* New York: Avon, 1976.

Kabat-Zinn, Jon. *Full Catastrophe Living.* New York: Dell, 1990.

Journal writing lowers stress levels and can be your best friend in the middle of the night when there's no one else to talk to. Write quickly, don't censor yourself, and find a safe place to keep your journal.

Resources:

Capacchione, Lucia. *The Well-Being Journal.* North Hollywood: Newcastle, 1989.

Remen, Rachel Naomi, M.D. *Kitchen Table Wisdom, Stories That Heal.* New York: Riverhead Books, 1996.

Creative art forms (painting, drawing, music, dance, poetry) are healing because you work with symbols and images to express feelings.

Resource: Capacchione, Lucia. *The Creative Journal.* North Hollywood: Newcastle, 1989.

Guided imagery is a specific kind of relaxation and movement using the mind's own images. Most mental health professionals who deal with illness can assist you in creating an individual tape that works for you. A prerequisite is to practice relaxation so you can access guided imagery. The technique uses all five senses and works best when it's tailored to you. Not everyone sees images, for example. If that's the case with you, the therapist will use sounds or smells instead.

Even if you don't hold formal religious beliefs, you can tap into your spirituality, says Pate-Willig. "Think back to your feelings at the birth of your child, or when you suddenly came upon a bed of glorious wild-flowers. Spirituality connects you with a sense of something larger than the self."

I appreciate every day since my liver transplant. I appreciate little things—like my morning glory plant. It's the most regal dark blue plant you ever saw, but it was dying.

I put that plant down in my little "hospital" under my deck, and this morning he had eight dark purple blossoms and new leaves. A little nurturing and he's back. I'm happier than if someone had given me money!

In 1996, I had an acute attack of hepatitis B, my liver failed, and I went into a coma. The Lord sure got my attention.

In the deepest part of the coma, it looked like I was floating to the brightest light I ever saw in my life. It was gorgeous—like going into a beautiful sun. I started drifting back. It got darker. And I woke up.

After the coma, I didn't know how to walk or talk. My hand coordination was bad. But now I think I'm made over. My eyes are white as snow, and my skin is clear.

When you come close to death, you're in God's hands. At church, they call me the miracle patient.

Illness, however, can also present a theological challenge. According to Dr. House, some patients "go through a crisis of faith. People who've gone to church all their lives may suddenly feel rejected, alone and abandoned, angry with God, or feel this illness is punishment for some unknown sin. Their social network is centered on their church, so if they lose this, they lose a lot. I recommend that they talk to their clergy or to the hospital chaplain."

"Spiritual distress," says Rev. Julie Swaney, Chaplain at the University of Colorado Health Sciences Center, "occurs when a person's faith or spirit is suddenly full of holes. Everything you believe in is gone. You've lost your value system, and you feel alone. But one of the gifts of illness is the way it opens us up to life. People reassess relationships, values, their sense of time, of what's important. Spirituality has to do with how we make meaning out of our experiences. Embrace what works for you."

Resources:

Benson, Herbert, M.D., with Marg Stark. *Timeless Healing, The Power and Biology of Belief.* New York: Scribner, 1996.

Byock, Ira, M.D. *Dying Well, Peace and Possibilities at the End of Life.* New York: Riverhead Books, 1997.

Frankl, Victor E. *Man's Search for Meaning.* New York: Simon & Schuster, 1984.

Kushner, Harold S. *When All You've Ever Wanted Isn't Enough.* New York: Simon & Schuster, 1986.

Moyers, Bill. *Healing and the Mind.* New York: Doubleday, 1993.

Finally, one last word on being good to yourself: Take small steps to wellness slowly, over time. There is no correct formula. You may move back and forth, concentrating first on one area, then another—whatever works!

There is no grief which time does not lessen and soften.

Cicero

Reference

[1] David Spiegel, M.D. *Living Beyond Limits.* (New York: Random House, 1993), p. 79.

7

TAKING CARE OF YOURSELF FINANCIALLY

An Overview

When I was diagnosed with hepatitis B twenty years ago, I experienced my first financial difficulties. I was living alone, self-employed, and very sick. I had no health insurance, and I was so ill I couldn't work for almost three months.

Things began to snowball. I got behind on my house payments and taxes. There was no end in sight, and I never did recover from my debts. My house went into foreclosure, and I wound up in bankruptcy.

Eventually, I made a career change and got back on track. With my new job I had medical insurance and short-term disability insurance. I was making plenty—but my hepatitis became chronic, and I had to take medical leave when I had flare-ups. At least this time I was covered!

Tim

LIKE TIM, you may feel too sick to work, but you can't quit because you need to hold on to your health insurance. Or you have so many medical bills, you're worried about paying the mortgage. Any chronic illness can put a dent in your budget.

Each one of you, however, faces a different situation. This chapter presents a general overview of financial issues and supplies you with resources to help you find your own solutions.*

We'll cover:

- Cost of Treatment
  Ongoing Medical Care
  Antiviral Treatment
  Transplantation
- Private Health Insurance
  Selecting Health Insurance
  Types of Private Health Insurance: Managed Care or Fee-for-Service
    HMOs
    PPOs
    Fee-for-Service Plans
- Government Health Insurance
  Medicare
  Medicaid
  Veterans Administration
- When You're Too Sick to Work: Applying for Disability
  Short-Term Disability Leave
- Disability Insurance
  Social Security Disability Insurance (SSDI)
  Supplemental Security Income (SSI)

Cost of Treatment

Ongoing Medical Care Costs. If you have a chronic illness, like hepatitis B, you have to consider the cost of lifelong medical care. At the very least, you need regular exams and blood tests to monitor your liver functions. For stable patients, the minimum recommendation is an annual physical examination and blood tests twice a year. You may also need a liver biopsy every three to five years. Ask your doctor what he or she recommends.

---

*Note: *This chapter is an overview, not an exhaustive treatment of financial options and programs. It does not provide legal advice; always contact agencies and companies for specific information and consult a lawyer for legal advice in specific cases.*

In the past year I've had a liver biopsy and a blood-clotting problem that landed me in the emergency room and intensive care unit overnight. That cost big time.

I've got health insurance, so I didn't worry until I heard that some insurance companies put a $1 million lifetime cap on their policies. It seemed like a fortune until I started to add up just this year's medical expenses. I finally called my company and found out my cap is $2 million. What a relief!

Susie

Antiviral Treatment Costs. At the time of this writing, three FDA-approved antiviral medications are available for the treatment of hepatitis B: interferon alpha-2b (INTRON® A), lamivudine (EPIVIR-HBV®), and Hepatitis B Immune Globulin (Nabi-HBV®, BayHep B®). Two other brands of interferon approved for hepatitis C treatment have not been FDA-approved specifically for hepatitis B. Your doctor, however, may choose to prescribe them: ROFERON®-A and INFERGEN®. In addition, the FDA approved pegylated interferon alpha-2b (PEG-INTRON™, Schering-Plough) for hepatitis C in January 2001. Pegylated interferon alpha-2a (PEGASYS®, Roche) awaits FDA approval at the time of this writing.

Call your health insurance provider to find out how much of the cost the provider will absorb. Expense depends on dosage or duration of therapy. Remember to budget for blood tests and doctors' visits to monitor your progress on treatment.

> **Resource:** For information about INTRON® A and PEG-INTRON™, call Schering-Plough at 1-800-222-7579 (website: www.schering.com).
>
> Schering's Commitment to Care℠ program (1-800-521-7157) offers help in finding coverage, cost-sharing, and the providing of drugs to indigent people. Have this information ready when you call:
> 1. name and address of your prescribing physician
> 2. diagnosis, prescribed drug therapy, and schedule
> 3. financial information: recent 1040 form, pay stub, Social Security number

Resource: For information on ROFERON®-A and PEGASYS®, call Roche customer service at 1-800-526-0625 (Website: www.rocheusa.com).

If you need help to pay for treatment, your doctor may contact Roche ONCOLINE Reimbursement Assistance Program: 1-800-443-6676.

Resource: For information on INFERGEN®, call Amgen customer service at 1-888-508-8088 (website: www.amgen.com).

INFERGEN® users who need financial aid to pay for the medication may call Amgen's SAFETY NET® Program at the COMPASS™ SUPPORT LINE: 1-888-508-8088.

Lamivudine, called EPIVIR-HBV®, comes in liquid or tablet form and is manufactured by GlaxoWellcome Inc.

Resource: For information on EPIVIR-HBV®, call the Glaxo Wellcome Customer Response Center, 1-888-825-5249 (TALK-2-GW). Website: www.glaxowellcome.com

If you need help paying for EPIVIR-HBV®, ask your health care advocate to call Glaxo Wellcome Patient Assistance Program at 1-800-722-9294.

Hepatitis B Immune Globulin (HBIG) provides immediate short-term protection against exposure to hepatitis B and post-transplant protection to prevent recurrence of the virus. Your doctor will order this medication for you. According to the Hepatitis B Foundation Drug Watch (February 2001), two companies' products are FDA-approved, Nabi and Bayer.

Resource: For an informative booklet titled *Take Action,* contact Nabi® Customer Operations at 1-800-458-4244. Websites: www.nabi.com and www.bayer.com

As of this writing, adefovir dipivoxil, developed by Gilead Sciences, is in the process of Phase III clinical trials.

Resource: Gilead Sciences Website: www.gilead.com

To keep up with the latest information on drugs either approved by the FDA or in development, contact the following:

Resource: The Hepatitis B Foundation compiles the *HBF Drug Watch* list: Hepatitis B Foundation, 700 East Butler Ave., Doylestown, PA 18901, 215-489-4900. Website: www.hepb.org

Resource: Contact the FDA at 1-888-INFO-FDA. Website: www.fda.gov

You might also consider enrolling in a study. Pharmaceutical companies often sponsor studies of promising new treatments; in many cases, the sponsor covers all costs of treatment. Be sure you understand exactly what the study involves, before you sign up for it. Ask your doctor for information or call a major research center or medical school near you (see Chapter 8, Treatment, and Chapter 13, Research Trends).

Transplantation Costs. The hospital's financial coordinator will be on your transplant team to help you figure out how you can afford the procedure. There are many costs involved: tests and consultations before the operation, the transplant operation itself, hospitalization, and follow-up care and medications.

> *Transplant coordinators are your best friends. They know how to research programs that give discounted or free medications, financial aid, and they know almost everyone in the hospital. My coordinator even talked to the hospital committee about the bills I couldn't pay because things got so critical for me financially.*
>
> Jerome

According to Fabi Imo, Coordinator, Transplant Financial Services at the University of Colorado Health Sciences Center, the cost for liver transplantation (from admission to discharge, but not including before or after care) varies widely, from $50,000 to more than $1 million. The average cost is approximately $150,000. Costs vary widely around the country.

Financial help is available. In December 1999, the Health Care Financing Administration (now known as the Centers for Medicare and Medicaid Services) reversed its policy against coverage for hepatitis B–related transplantation and announced that Medicare would cover the costs of liver transplants for hepatitis B patients. In addition, "Transplantation and living donor liver transplantation are more accepted medical procedures now so they are covered by more insurance companies," says

Imo. "Presently, Medicare and our state of Colorado Medicaid approve living donor transplantation because it is no longer considered an experimental procedure.

"Work with your hospital transplant financial coordinator to consider all your options. People often have insurance benefits they're not aware of. For example, some patients are covered for travel, lodging, and mileage costs."

According to Imo, sometimes patients who need financial help find themselves in a "Catch-22" situation. If you are disabled by liver disease and apply for Social Security Disability Insurance, a federal program, it takes 24 months (starting from the date you became eligible) for Medicare to become effective. Medicare does pay for liver transplants, but you may not be in a condition to wait two years.

"Another 'Catch-22' situation is the biggest problem I see," says Imo. "If the patient is over the minimum eligibility level, he or she will not qualify for Medicaid. And even if you have Medicaid, not all state Medicaid programs will cover a liver transplant. Colorado Medicaid will cover the transplant for hepatitis B patients, but Wyoming, Nebraska, and Montana Medicaid, for example, do not cover the procedure for patients over the age of 21."

Not all private insurance policies cover transplants, and both private and government health insurance impose certain criteria. For example, people who have additional medical problems, such as a heart condition, a malignancy, or HIV, may find themselves excluded from coverage.

> At first my insurance company wouldn't cover the transplant because I had gone on new insurance the year before. They said my liver disease was a pre-existing condition, but my husband persisted.
>
> "If she knew she was sick and didn't reveal it," he told them, "that's grounds to not pay. But she always showed up for work, and no one knew she was sick." The company agreed to pay.
>
> *Lila*

In addition to determining insurance coverage for the transplant procedure itself, it's also important to look at your prescription drug benefit and how it covers immunosuppressive drugs. According to Imo, "The medications probably are the largest financial expense out of the patient's pocket. Post-transplant immunosuppressive medicines can be thousands of dollars a month." If you need help with medication costs, talk to your transplant coordinator about possible resources, such as pharmaceutical companies and other organizations.

Note: Medicare recently eliminated its former three-year time limit for coverage of post-transplant immunosuppressive medicines and now pays 80 percent of immunosuppressive drug costs for the lifetime of the transplanted organ. This policy applies to all Medicare-entitled beneficiaries who meet all of the other program requirements for coverage under this benefit.

Adding to direct costs are many indirect expenses. Patients sometimes forget to allow for organ recovery costs or travel and lodging for family members, child care, and so on. It's important to plan ahead.

Finally, cautions Imo, it's important for patients to be involved with insurance companies. Know the name and phone number of your case manager, and always inform your financial coordinator and your liver transplant team immediately if you change insurance companies.

Resource: A 48-page booklet by the United Network for Organ Sharing (UNOS) discusses a number of topics, including financing transplantation. It includes a list of organizations that provide help for transplant expenses, such as Children's Organ Transplant Association (COTA®) and the National Foundation for Transplants (formerly Organ Transplant Fund). For a copy of *What Every Patient Needs to Know,* call 1-888-TXINFO1 (1-888-894-6361). The book also appears on the UNOS Website: www.unos.org

Resource: Another booklet, written by volunteers and distributed by the Organ Donor Program, may be helpful. For your free copy of *Finger in the Dike, Or: How to Raise $140,000 for Organ Transplant Surgery in Less Than Four Weeks,* call 1-800-452-1369 and ask for the Organ Donor Program.

Resource: The American Liver Foundation (ALF) has established a Liver Transplant Fund that provides professional administration, at no cost, for funds raised on behalf of patients to help pay for medical care and associated transplantation expenses. They also offer a pamphlet on fundraising suggestions. For information, call 1-800-GO-LIVER or 1-888-4-HEP-ABC.

Private Health Insurance

When I sold my business, I knew I had to get some good medical insurance because I was feeling really bad. I applied for a job with a big national company. They said, "You're overqualified. Do you really want to do this?" I said yes—and picked up 100 percent insurance coverage. A caseworker from the company called to say she'd be handling my case, and if I did have the transplant, it would be covered with no deductible!

Sometimes I say, "Why me?" Other times I say this is a payback for straightening my life out. I have this belief that I'm going to be okay, and things will work out as they should.

Caroline

Selecting Private Health Insurance. When you have a chronic illness like hepatitis B, you must select your health insurance carefully:

- Read your policy before signing it. Ask questions. If there is any part you don't understand, get help.
- Make sure your plan allows you to see doctors who are experts in hepatitis B: gastroenterologists, hepatologists, and transplant physicians.
- Understand the restrictions and make sure they won't affect the quality of your care. For example, does the policy cover emergency rooms, experimental treatments, drugs like interferon? What happens if you're out of town and you need medical help?
- Is there a lifetime limit or cap on treatment or drugs? A million dollars may sound high, but is it too low for a chronic condition?
- Use common sense in assessing a medical policy. When you have hepatitis B, you have to plan ahead for extra medical care, even though you may never need it.
- Check to see if your policy pays based on "reasonable and customary" fee schedules. Policies that use fee schedules may not pay the entire bill if they feel that your doctor or hospital does not charge "reasonable" rates.
- Know any managed care provisions in your policy. Do you have any particular doctor or hospital that you are required to use? If you use a "preferred provider," will the insurance cover a larger share?

Types of Private Health Insurance: Managed Care or Fee-for-Service. Private health insurance policies fall into two categories:

(1) managed care, or (2) fee for service. Managed care plans limit your choice of physician, but usually cost less. Managed care options include Health Maintenance Organizations (HMO) and Preferred Provider Organizations (PPO).

Fee-for-service policies usually provide the freedom to choose your doctor, but they often are more expensive. Look at the following factors when comparing cost of fee-for-service policies:

- monthly premiums—what the insurance costs each month
- annual deductible—how much you have to pay out of your pocket each year before the policy will pay benefits
- co-insurance—what percentage you have to pay that your insurance will not cover, usually 20 to 30 percent
- out-of-pocket maximum—the amount that you pay in co-insurance before the insurance company will begin to pay at 100 percent
- policy maximum—the maximum amount that insurance will pay over the lifetime of the policy

Whether you choose a managed care or traditional fee-for-service plan, be sure you understand how your plan works and the appeal process. If you're dissatisfied with your insurance policy, you may always review these issues with your State Commissioner of Insurance.

HMOs. Under HMO plans you have a primary care physician, a gate-keeper, who coordinates your care and decides if you should be referred to a specialist. This plan is the least costly but the most limiting in terms of freedom of choice. Because the goal is to keep costs at a minimum, your access to specialists, tests, medications, or hospital care may be restricted. It's important to do a thorough check on limitations.

PPOs. You may choose a doctor within the provider network and get 90 to 100 percent coverage of your costs or choose a doctor outside the network and receive a smaller percentage of the cost, usually 70 percent.

Fee-for-Service Plans. Usually, the choice of doctor is totally yours, but these plans are typically the most expensive. Patients with chronic hepatitis B who are exploring fee-for-service plans should choose a major medical policy that offers subspecialty physician services and ade-quate hospital coverage.

The insurance company usually pays 80 percent of the bill, and you pay 20 percent up to a total amount designated by your policy. Hospital and physician fees that the insurance company deems unreasonable may not be fully reimbursed.

Resource: To help consumers with the process of choosing a suitable health-care plan, check out two government Websites: The Quality Inter-agency Coordination Task Force (a group of federal agencies involved with health care) at www.consumer.gov/qualityhealth/in dex.html and the Department of Health and Human Services at www.healthfinder.gov/smartchoices/qualitycare/default.htm.

Resource: For help in evaluating health insurance plans, call the National Committee for Quality Assurance at 1-800-839-6487 for a personalized list of accredited HMOs in your area or visit their Web-site to view *Choosing Quality: Finding the Health Plan That's Right for You* (archives section): www.ncqa.org.

Resource: Another useful booklet is *Checkup on Health Insurance Choices*, AHCPR #93-0018, by the Agency for Health Care Policy and Research: 1-800-358-9295.

Resource: In 1996, Congress passed the Health Insurance Portability and Accountability Act (Public Law #104-191), sponsored by Senators Edward Kennedy and Nancy Kassebaum. This act includes many significant health insurance reforms.

Some highlights of the act include: (1) "portability" provisions, (2) increased availability of coverage, and (3) expansion of COBRA continuation coverage benefits. The "portability" provisions are designed to eliminate the fear that employees will lose their health insurance if they change jobs.

You may request a copy of the act and its accompanying conference committee report from your U.S. representative or senator. Also, as with other legislation of this type, government agencies, such as the Labor Department, the Internal Revenue Service, and the Department of Health and Human Services, will issue regulations to implement the act's provisions. In addition, almost all states will have to make changes in state legislation to comply with the act. For information, call your state legislators and your state insurance department.

Resource: Some states have set up risk-sharing pools to enable people who are otherwise uninsurable to purchase health insurance. Colorado, for example, has the Colorado Uninsurable Health Insurance Plan (CUHIP). State insurance laws differ, so call your state insurance department for specific information. If you have difficulty locating your state insurance department, contact the National Association of Insurance Commissioners for the listing: 816-842-3600. Website: www.naic.org

Government Health Insurance

Caution: Laws and regulations change over time. Double-check your facts with the agency involved. Only the agency itself can give you up-to-date, accurate material.

There are some situations when Medicare may eventually end, based on Social Security Disability Insurance (SSDI) eligibility. Also, the effects of work on benefits [SSDI and Supplemental Security Income (SSI)] and Medicare/Medicaid are complicated and different depending on what benefit you get. The best thing to do is to call the Social Security Administration at 1-800-772-1213 before you or your spouse works to see what the specific effects will be on your cash benefits and/or medical coverage.

This chapter does not give legal advice and is not a substitute for the professional services of an attorney. Always consult a lawyer when legal issues are involved.

Medicare. At age 65, you may be eligible for medical insurance for hospital and other medical services. If you are entitled to Social Security disability benefits for 24 consecutive months (see following section), you also may qualify for Medicare.

Medicare has two parts. Hospital insurance (Part A) covers inpatient hospital care. You already paid for this as part of your Social Security and Medicare taxes when you were working. Medical insurance (Part B) pays for doctors' services, prescriptions, and some outpatient facility and doctor visits. Part B is optional, and you'll be billed monthly for your premium.

If you are not already getting Social Security benefits, sign up for Medicare at your local Social Security office three months before you become 65, and you'll receive your Medicare card. Ask about enrollment periods. If you are getting Social Security benefits, you will automatically be enrolled, and you will receive your card in the mail. You may also want to purchase a Medigap policy, or HMO, or other Medicare supplement (private insurance that fills in some of the "gaps" in Medicare's coverage).

Resources: Call the Centers for Medicare and Medicaid Services (CMS) Medicare Hotline (1-800-638-6833) or access its Website (www.medicare.gov) to order publications, such as the *Medicare & You* handbook, and to get more information on Medigap supplemental insurance.

If you have a low income and few resources, you may qualify for state aid to help pay for Medicare premiums and some other expenses; ask for CMS's *Guide to Health Insurance*. You may also call the Department of Social Services.

Medicaid. Medicaid is a federal-state health program for people with low assets and incomes. At present, the program is administered by state social services departments. To apply, call your county social services department.

Veterans Administration (VA). For questions about medical benefits and disability, veterans may call the Veterans Administration Regional Office.

> *I found out that being in the armed forces, I was eligible for benefits through the VA hospital. With disability as my only source of income, I could get my medical needs met for free—no co-pays, no out-of-pocket payments for procedures—and all my medications cost me $2 each. When I switched to the VA hospital for care, I still maintained my time accrued on the national transplant list.*
>
> *All I had to do was provide them with a copy of my DD214 proving I was a veteran and a copy of my eligibility papers from Social Security. The whole process took me 15 minutes.*
>
> *Arthur*

Resource: Dial this number and your call will be automatically directed to your regional VA office: 1–800–827–1000.

When You're Too Sick to Work: Applying for Disability

As hepatitis B progresses to the stage of cirrhosis, you may be less capable of functioning at home or on the job. In general, this occurs only in patients who have had the disease for many years and who have cirrhosis and signs of worsening liver function.

Our goal in this section is to provide you with a general overview of the available options for disability benefits and the process involved. For those who wish to consider applying for disability benefits, the process varies depending on your income, personal situation, and insurers or government programs.

Caution:
1. Laws and regulations change; unexpected circumstances arise. It's best to double-check your facts with the company, agency, or organization involved. Medical social workers can help direct you to the appropriate agencies or programs.
2. Keep a file with copies of all your medical records. Begin right now, if you haven't already done so. Always keep your Explanation of Benefit (EOB) forms sent to you by your insurance company. The EOB is the document that explains what the medical provider and/or hospital is paid and contains a description of payment procedures.
3. Start a journal. Keep track of your symptoms and how they affect your daily tasks. This documentation will help you explain your symptoms to your doctor and will be important later if you ever have to file for disability.
4. This chapter does not give legal advice and is not a substitute for the professional services of an attorney. Consider consultation with a lawyer when legal issues or hearings are involved.

Resource: Call the American Bar Association at 312-988-5000 for your state's lawyer referral service number or check your phone book. Attorneys specialize in different areas, such as disability or insurance, so explain your specific problem.

If you can't afford a lawyer, contact your local Legal Aid Society or a law school that sponsors a student association offering free legal advice. Your local United Way may also direct you to possible sources of legal help.

Short-Term Disability Leave. Become familiar with your company's policies. Some companies offer paid short-term disability leave or allow you to use accumulated sick days. Companies usually require that a doctor accurately assess the nature of your symptoms and verify that you are disabled. The diagnosis of hepatitis B or treatment with interferon and other antiviral medications are not sufficient, in and of themselves, to necessarily justify disability.

If you are an eligible employee and you or your family member (child, parent, spouse) becomes seriously ill from advanced hepatitis B, the Family and Medical Leave Act allows you to take up to 12 weeks of unpaid leave each year. Workers returning from leave must be restored to their original jobs or equivalent jobs with the same pay, benefits, and working conditions.

In 1997, while returning from a business trip, I had a major medical emergency and was rushed to the hospital. This time it was serious. I was in the hospital for almost six weeks. They told me I needed a liver transplant.

I was able to continue working for a while, but over the next year-and-a-half my energy level dropped significantly. I couldn't work for more than 20 hours a month. At that point, I had to take advantage of the Family and Medical Leave Act to try to recuperate. Taking 12 weeks of unpaid medical leave ate up my financial resources pretty quickly.

Samantha

Resource: For more information and to find out if you are an eligible employee under the act, call the nearest office of the Wage and Hour Division, listed in most telephone directories under U.S. Government, Department of Labor, Employment Standards Administration. Ask for copies of these publications: WH Publication #1420, Your Rights *Under the Family and Medical Leave Act,* WH Publication #1421, *Compliance Guide to the Family and Medical Leave Act,* U.S. Department of Labor, Wage and Hour Division, Dec. 1996, and Fact Sheet No. ESA 93-24, U.S. Department of Labor Program Highlights, *The Family and Medical Leave Act of 1993.*

Resource: The 1990 Americans with Disabilities Act (ADA) prohibits job discrimination against "qualified individuals with disabilities." Employers covered under the act must make a "reasonable accommodation" for such persons depending on the particular facts in each case and on whether or not it imposes "due hardship" on the employer. "Reasonable accommodations" apply to the area of attendance and leave policies. To see if the ADA covers you and your employer and to get more specific information on the provisions of the act, call the President's Committee on Employment of People with Disabilities Job Accommodation Network) at 1-800-ADA-WORK or 1-800-526-7234. Email: jan@jan.icdi.wvu.edu. Website: www.jan.wvu.edu

Disability Insurance

If you're self-employed, you may have paid for your own individual disability insurance. If you work for a company, find out if you are eligible to enroll in your company's group disability coverage. Read the terms of coverage carefully.

> *When I went on disability, I was at my highest earning capacity. It's a good thing I couldn't take a less stressful job at my company for less money. I would have had to quit anyway, and then I would have shot myself in the foot because my disability was computed as a percentage of my paycheck. It's hard enough to live on what I did get—60 percent of what I was earning.*
>
> *Jenny*

> *When they told me I had cirrhosis from hepatitis B and needed to be on the transplant list, I thought, "Oh, oh, oh—what, what, what. This is serious. Transplants are what happen to other people."*
>
> *The bill was $125,000 for the doctors and hospital. I paid zero. I have fantastic insurance here at work.*
>
> *Larry*

Two Social Security Administration programs offer assistance if you have to file for disability: Social Security Disability Insurance (SSDI) and Supplemental Security Income (SSI).

Caution: Brief descriptions of the programs follow, but only the agency itself can give you up-to-date, accurate material. *Call the Social Security Administration and ask them to send you information about disability programs: 1-800-772-1213.* You can speak to a service representative between the hours of 7 a.m. and 7 p.m. on business days. Hearing-impaired callers using TTY equipment can call 1-800-325-0778 during the same hours.

Social Security Disability Insurance (SSDI). This insurance covers workers (and their children or surviving spouses). In order to qualify for this disability coverage on your own record, you must have worked long enough and recently enough to have made sufficient contributions to your Social Security account. You may also qualify on the record of a parent or as a disabled widow(er). Adults must have a physical and/or mental problem that prevents them from working for at least a year or that is expected to result in death. Benefits continue until a person is able to work and earn a certain amount of money again on a regular basis.

You may file a claim by phone, mail, or by visiting the nearest Social Security office. The claims process can take about 180 days while the agency obtains medical information and decides if the disability affects your ability to work. You'll be asked to provide your Social Security number and proof of age and citizenship; names, addresses, and phone numbers of doctors, hospitals, clinics, and institutions that treated you and dates of treatment; names of all medications you are taking; medical records from your doctors, therapists, hospitals, clinics, and caseworkers; laboratory and test results; a summary of where you worked in the past 15 years and the kind of work you did; a copy of your W-2 Form (Wage and Tax Statement), or if you are self-employed, your federal tax return for the past year; dates of prior marriages if your spouse is applying.

Social Security will request medical records from your physicians and hospitals to document your disability. However, your application will be processed faster if you provide this information for them up front when you apply.

The Social Security Administration recommends that you don't wait to file your claim, even if you don't have all this information right away. (There is a waiting period before benefits begin, so the sooner you apply, the better.) If you need someone's help, a family member, caseworker, or other representative can contact the agency for you.

After your application is complete, the Social Security office will review it to see if you're eligible. Then they'll send your application to the Disability Determination Services (DDS) office in your state. (Consult SSA Publication No. 05-10029, which lists five questions that determine disability.)

If the claim is approved, you'll receive a notice showing the amount of your benefit and when payments start. The amount of your benefit is based on your lifetime average earnings covered by Social Security, but workers' compensation benefits can affect your disability check. Your case will be reviewed periodically to see if you remain disabled. After two years from the date of first eligibility of disability, you will be eligible for Medicare benefits, regardless of your age. If your claim is denied, a notice will explain why, and you will have opportunities to contest the decision.

Here are some patients' stories:

First, I had to go to Social Services to apply for temporary assistance and food stamps while Social Security was processing my application, which I was told could take up to three months. I was granted temporary assistance. That gave me $300 per month and $125 for food stamps. Needless to say, this was not a whole lot to live on. It didn't even cover my rent, much less utilities, telephone, or insurance co-payments.

I had to do a lot of paperwork, such as getting letters from doctors, filling out applications, and doing follow-up. I feel very fortunate that I was given lots of special treatment and cooperation from Social Services, Social Security, and my doctors.

So how did I make it this far? Here is a tip. Ask for help, whether it's financial help from family and friends or help to be your voice when you just don't have the energy to do it yourself.

I keep records of all the people I talk to, what their job is, and I get their first and last names and phone numbers. If I ask for this information, they know that I'm going to follow up with them, and they will be motivated to work on my problem. Also, if I'm not feeling well enough to take care of stuff, my family will have the list.

Once I was on disability, money was short. I found out that I could apply for a program through the public utility company that pays my heating bill during the winter. It was a one-page application, and it only took five minutes to fill out. That saves me $400 a year—and I need the money for meds. I also found out that the local phone company had a program that paid for my basic service. This was handled with one phone call and saved me another $200 a year.

Here I am—no energy, no resources, and stressing about how do I have a life. Sometimes I have even found myself sitting at home alone during the day and asking myself if I can make it through—and I'm not one that gives up easily! It's important to remember that there are always options.

I was so sick. The pain was indescribable. I was fatigued, and I lost my concentration. I couldn't remember the codes at work anymore. They didn't soak in. Finally, the doctor said it was time to stop work.

I filled out all the disability forms, explained my situation, and was denied. I got an attorney, appealed, and was denied. I had to go before an administrative judge, and I got it based on my depression—not on my liver disease.

I had five psych evaluations in three years, and they all agreed I was depressed. I have been treated since 1992 when I saw a liver doctor who asked me if I was suicidal. I had figured out how I would do it with the meds I had, but I had not consciously realized I had done this, and it scared me to death. That's when I started on anti-depressants.

While I was fighting Workman's Comp and Social Security, I was on disability and receiving 60 percent of my pay. I had no health insurance because the premiums cost $500 a month, and I couldn't afford that.

Two days after my insurance ran out, one of my kids broke his arm. I'll be paying for it until he goes to college. You could lose everything you have while waiting for Social Security—and then you have to wait some more.

It makes me sad because I've worked since I was 16 years old. It hurts my feelings when people say I'm lazy. I've worked hard all my life to care for the people around me, and now I have to fight for every penny.

Once you've had a bleed, Social Security disability is no problem at all. It's life-threatening. I couldn't believe it. All my friends told me it would take months, and I got disability in seven weeks!

Later, after the bleed and after my husband was admitted to the hospital, I started thinking of myself and the kids. This financial stuff affects the spouse.

Both the boys were in college. One had to get a loan. I had to drop my master's program. Tom is a hard worker, and he couldn't stand it. It was hard on him.

When he appied for disability, they made us wait six months before we saw any money. You can't even apply before you do a godawful amount of paperwork. I said to the clerk, "Why does he have to wait six months? We put the money in, and we can't get it back when we need it. Is this so you can give him time to pass away so you don't have to pay?"

Hepatitis B can take a financial toll on your life. It was a big adjustment for me to go from $80,000 a year to $984 a month, especially when rent is $500 and meds are $300.

You have to tap into other resources. You have to do things you don't want to do, like reach out to family. It's hard. Fortunately, my family has been good about helping me out.

Resource: Call the Social Security Administration at 1-800-772-1213 (Website: http://www.ssa.gov) for copies of SSA Publication No. 05-10057, *Social Security Disability Programs Can Help;* SSA Publication No. 05-10029, *Social Security Disability Benefits;* SSA Publication No. 05-10153, *What You Need to Know When You Get Disability Benefits;* SSA Publication No. 05-10041, *The Appeals Process;* SSA Publication No. 05-10075, Your Right to Representation.

Resource: Jehle, Faustin F. *The Complete & Easy Guide to Social Security, Healthcare Rights & Government Benefits.* Boca Raton: Emerson–Adams Press, 1998.

Resource: Mathews, Joseph L. with Dorothy Berman. *Social Security, Medicare, and Pensions.* Berkeley: Nolo.com. 1999.

Supplemental Security Income (SSI). SSI is a Social Security Administration program that makes disability payments to adults and children with little or no income or resources. To get SSI, you must be 65 or older, or blind or disabled. According to SSA Publication No. 05-11000, *Supplemental Security Income,* disabled means you have a physical or mental problem that keeps you from substantial work and is expected to last at least a year or to result in death.

The basic SSI payment is the same all over the country, but some states add money to your check. Any income you or your spouse has may affect the check amount. Call the Social Security Administration for information.

It's hard to go on disability, but I was fortunate to work with a social worker who hand-walked my file all the way through. I've been on disability for 14 months now. At 24 months, I will qualify for Medicare and Medicaid.

When I was so sick, I got disability payments. I felt guilty taking the money because I have a strong work ethic. So I made up my mind I would contribute to society—and I do—by helping with a support group for people with hepatitis B.

If you qualify for SSI, in most states you will be able to get other aid from your state or county, such as Medicaid (which helps pay doctor and hospital bills), food stamps, or other social services. Call your local social services department or public welfare office.

If you get Medicare and have low income and few resources, you may qualify for help with some Medicare premiums or co-pays under the Qualified Medicare Beneficiary (QMB) or Specified Low-Income Medicare Beneficiary (SLMB) programs. Only your state can decide if you qualify. Contact your county Social Services.

Whether your income meets SSI requirements depends on some very specific criteria defining what's included in income and what's included as assets outlined in SSA Publication No. 05-11000, *Supplemental Security Income.*

Sometimes people can get both Social Security and SSI benefits. The rules that determine if you're disabled are the same for Social Security and SSI (refer to the previous section, Social Security Disability Insurance). You must be unable to do any substantial kind of work to be considered disabled under both programs.

If you think you are eligible for SSI, the Social Security Administration recommends that you file a claim right away, even if you don't have all the information at hand. The information you need includes your Social Security card or a record of your Social Security number; your birth certificate or other proof of age; proof of citizenship; information about the home where you live (such as mortgage, lease, landlord's name); information about your income and the things you own (such as payroll slips, bank books, insurance policies, car registration, burial fund records, etc.), and names, addresses, and telephone numbers of doctors, hospitals, and clinics.

Resource: Call the Social Security Administration at 1-800-772-1213 (Website: http://www.ssa.gov). Hearing-impaired callers using TTY equipment, call 1-800-325-0778. Explain why you're calling and ask for helpful information and pamphlets, including SSA Publication No. 05-10057, *Social Security Disability Programs Can Help;* SSA Publication No. 05-11000, *Supplemental Security Income;* SSA Publication No. 05-10101, *Food Stamp Facts;* SSA Publication No. 05-10100, *Food Stamps And Other Nutrition Programs;* SSA Publication No. 05-11011, *What You Need to Know When You Get SSI;* and SSA Publication No. 05-11069, *You May Be Able to Get SSI.*

Resource: Jehle, Faustin F. *The Complete & Easy Guide to Social Security, Healthcare Rights & Government Benefits.* Boca Raton: Emerson-Adams Press. 1998.

Riches serve a wise man but command a fool.

English proverb

8

TREATMENT FOR HEPATITIS B

Interferon, Lamivudine, and Adefovir

I was eager to start interferon but had a poor response initially. My white count was low. It was pretty, pretty scary. I started with a dose of 5 million, but I had to drop to 3 million. The doctors didn't think it would work, but I did develop antibodies!

I was so psyched to succeed. I drew strength from everything—my religion, my family and friends. It was hard to handle something so unfair. But I'm a caretaker. I have two children, and I support my parents financially. The idea that I'd be gone from their lives—I just couldn't accept that.

Tammy

MAKING TREATMENT decisions can be a stressful process. You and your doctor will work together to decide on a treatment plan. But it helps to know as much as you can about your options.

In this chapter I'll cover the following topics:

- Overview: General Guidelines for Patients with Chronic Hepatitis B
    Treatment for Acute Hepatitis B
    Treatment for Chronic Hepatitis B
    Monitoring Patients with Chronic Infection
- Interferon
    What Is Interferon?
    Types of Interferon
    Pegylated Interferons
    Who Should Take Interferon?
    Interferon Monotherapy
    Prednisone "Priming" Followed by Interferon
    Interferon Plus Lamivudine
    Interferon Plus Ribavirin
    Measuring Response to Interferon Treatment
    Predictors of Response
    The Patient's Experience: Interferon Injections
    Interferon Side Effects
    Treatment Tips from Patients
- Lamivudine
    What Is Lamivudine (EPIVIR-HBV®)?
    Who Should Take Lamivudine?
    Measuring Response to Lamivudine Treatment
    Predictors of Response
    Pre-Core Mutation
    YMDD Mutations
    Side Effects
- Thymosin-alpha1 (Zadaxin®)
- Famciclovir (Famvir®) and Ganciclovir (Cytovene®)
    Side Effects
- Adefovir Dipivoxil
    What Is Adefovir?
    Who Should Take Adefovir?
    Measuring Response
    Side Effects
- After Treatment, What Next?
    If You Are a Nonresponder to Interferon Monotherapy
    If You Are a Nonresponder to Lamivudine

Overview: General Guidelines for Patients with Hepatitis B

As a patient with hepatitis B, you may experience fatigue, loss of energy, loss of concentrating ability, and a sense of inadequacy in performing your daily activities. These symptoms, feelings, and attitudes may make you emotional or susceptible to periods of depression.

If you are suffering an initial, acute attack, you have an excellent chance of recovering completely (see below, Treatment for Acute Hepatitis B, for more detailed guidelines). If you have chronic hepatitis B, I encourage you to continue to remain physically active, pursue your occupation, socialize, and maintain proper nutrition. I also recommend regular exercise and a well-balanced diet supplemented with 400 IU Vitamin E and one multivitamin per day. (See Chapters 5 and 6 for more detailed suggestions on how to take care of yourself nutritionally and emotionally.)

Remember: Alcohol and hepatitis B don't mix.   Avoid excessive alcohol intake; the combination of alcohol and hepatitis B may accelerate your liver disease. I discourage daily drinking or taking large amounts of alcohol at any time.

However, alcohol use is socially acceptable, so many patients ask me if they can take a drink once in a while. If you're not willing to abstain completely from alcohol, you should at least limit your alcohol intake to less than two ounces a week.

I had been a chronic alcohol drinker since I returned from Vietnam. Unfortunately, after my first attack of hepatitis B I didn't follow the doctor's advice about alcohol and continued to drink. Now I've stopped, but I've got cirrhosis.

Pete

Patients also question me about alternative therapies. A number of herbal remedies, teas, potions, and over-the-counter products claim to be effective in treating liver disease and viral hepatitis. Some of these therapies may ultimately prove useful, but at this time none have been adequately studied. The use of these treatments to eradicate hepatitis B is not encouraged because their effectiveness is doubtful and their safety, in general, is unknown. Be sure to check with your doctor before taking any over-the-counter products or other substances (see Chapter 5, Herbs Harmful to the Liver).

Treatment for Acute Hepatitis B. If you are suffering an initial, acute attack of hepatitis B, you may experience flu-like symptoms, abdominal discomfort, mild fever, headache, muscle pain, and even jaundice. Exteme fatigue is common with acute hepatitis B.

> *I started feeling a pain in my side and felt really rundown. I did not have the notion to do anything. Getting out of bed, walking across the room was an effort. I couldn't even drive the car to the grocery store. When I went to the bathroom, my urine was dark.*
>
> *Blood work showed I had hepatitis B. I told the doctor I felt pretty awful, but he said, "The only thing you can do is wait it out. We can't give you a shot or anything."*
>
> Ted

> *My 25-year-old son Jon, who's an athlete, got an acute attack of hepatitis B. He was badly jaundiced. The doctor told him off because when he started to feel a bit better, he played a little football and ran. Then he felt unwell again.*
>
> *He finally got it into his head that getting better would take time. It took a while for him to accept that he couldn't push himself. When he learned the signs of fatigue, he rested up.*
>
> *Gradually, month by month, his energy levels increased. His appetite is still not brilliant, but the doctor gave us good news on Friday. Jon doesn't have chronic hepatitis. He got the all clear!*
>
> Allison

People have a very high chance of recovering completely from an initial, acute attack. Approximately 90 to 95 percent of adults with acute hepatitis B recover and remain immune to re-infection throughout their lifetime.

Generally, you will be treated as an outpatient and monitored with blood tests and periodic assessment of your symptoms. You should take care to maintain adequate intake of fluids and calories and get plenty of rest. Specific treatments, such as interferon or lamivudine, are not used to treat acute hepatitis B.

Your doctor will watch for signs of liver failure—a rare event that occurs in only 0.1 to 1 percent of patients with acute hepatitis B. Symptoms of serious liver injury include severe jaundice, elevation in pro-thrombin (blood clotting) time, acidosis (a buildup of acids in the blood), renal (kidney) failure, or altered mental status. If you develop any of these signs, you may need to be hospitalized or referred to a center skilled in liver transplantation.

Close personal and household contacts of a patient with acute hepatitis B are at risk for infection. They should get hepatitis B immune globulin (HBIG) and hepatitis B vaccine to minimize this risk (see Vaccination and HBIG sections in this chapter).

Treatment for Chronic Hepatitis B. (See Figure 8A) Five to 10 percent of adults with acute infection fail to clear the virus and develop chronic infection. Chronic hepatitis B is diagnosed by the following:

- elevation in liver enzymes for more than six months
- markers of ongoing viral infection (HBsAg, eAg, and HBV DNA)
- liver biopsy demonstrating inflammation and fibrosis

If you have chronic hepatitis B, often you may not have symptoms, and your enzyme levels may be highly variable. Some patients have persistent mild to moderate elevations in liver enzymes. Others exhibit flares in activity with marked elevations in enzymes and even jaundice with intervening periods of normal or nearly normal enzyme activity. Flares in disease activity are typically accompanied by flu-like symptoms (poor appetite, lethargy, myalgia, headache, and low grade fever). Active inflammation in the setting of chronic hepatitis B is usually associated with evidence of active viral replication and positive surface antigen, e antigen, and HBV DNA.

After my first attack of hepatitis B, I went back to work. I continued to have pains in my liver. I stopped all alcohol, and I didn't have

FIGURE 8A: CURRENT OPTIONS FOR ANTIVIRAL THERAPY OF CHRONIC HEPATITIS B.

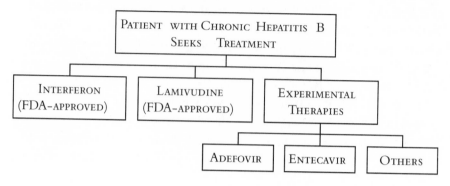

LEGEND 8A: The FDA currently has approved two treatments for chronic hepatitis B: interferon alfa-2b (INTRON® A, Schering-Plough) and lamivudine (EPIVIR-HBV®, Glaxo Wellcome). Adefovir dipivoxil and entecavir are in later stages of clinical investigation and may receive FDA approval in the near future. Others, such as nucleoside analogues, ribozymes, anti-sense molecules, and vaccines are under development, in preclinical study, or in the early phases of clinical investigation.

problems with my hepatitis for quite a while. Then I started to have flare-ups every three to four months.

I was antigen positive, definitely a carrier. My energy was much lower, and there'd be tenderness in the area around my liver. I became a strict vegetarian, and the flare-ups stopped. But three years ago, I found out I had cirrhosis.

Ron

Current criteria for treatment of patients with chronic hepatitis B with either interferon or lamivudine include:

- abnormal ALT
- positive eAg
- positive HBV DNA

Both treatments have their advocates. Doctors who favor the use of interferon as first-line therapy point to the 25 to 40 percent chance to clear the virus and remain free of infection. Those who favor the use of lamivudine as first-line therapy emphasize the lack of side effects (few with lamivudine vs. many with interferon) and ease of administration (pills for lamivudine vs. injection for interferon). In addition, in some studies the chance for long-term viral clearance post-treatment was the same for both interferon and lamivudine.

In this chapter we discuss both interferon and lamivudine in detail, list the advantages and disadvantages of each, and review experience with other agents (thymosin-alpha1, famciclovir, ganciclovir). Other topics of interest to patients being treated for chronic infection include the management of both renal disease and polyarteritis nodosa due to hepatitis B (see Chapter 3). We will also cover an emerging problem, the YMDD mutation, and focus discussion on new and developing therapies, such as adefovir dipivoxil.

Monitoring Patients with Chronic Infection. There are two types of chronic infection: the chronic carrier without evidence of liver disease and the patient with chronic hepatitis B.

Chronic carriers who acquired the infection as newborns via transmission from their infected mothers are at risk for developing liver cancer and should be monitored for this life-threatening complication. Typical monitoring procedures include assessment of alpha-fetoprotein (blood test) and ultrasonography of the liver every six months. Chronic carriers who acquired the infection in adult life are less at risk for liver cancer, and screening is not recommended until they have the infection for more than 20 years.

Patients with chronic hepatitis B need to be monitored for both progression to cirrhosis and liver cancer. Factors that predict progression to cirrhosis include active inflammation and fibrosis on liver biopsy, excessive intake of alcohol, excessive iron accumulation in the liver, and co-infection with delta agent, hepatitis C, or HIV.

The risk of liver cancer is particularly increased in patients with chronic hepatitis who develop cirrhosis. Recent data indicate that the risk of liver cancer in cirrhotics with hepatitis B is comparable to the risk in cirrhotics with hepatitis C—about 2 percent per year. We recommend screening for liver cancer every six months for patients with chronic hepatitis B who have cirrhosis (see Chapter 10).

Interferon

What Is Interferon? Scientists identified interferon in 1957 by demonstrating that cells infected with a virus secrete a substance that has the ability to protect other uninfected cells from becoming infected. This substance, interferon, is a naturally occurring protein whose name is derived from its ability to interfere with viral replication.

Types of Interferon. Since these early studies, the interferon story has become increasingly complex with three currently recognized classes of interferons: alpha, beta, and gamma. In treating hepatitis B, gamma interferon is ineffective, and beta interferon is less effective than alpha interferon. Alpha interferons are the most effective interferons for treatment of hepatitis B.

Interferon-alfa-2b (INTRON® A, Schering-Plough) is currently the only interferon approved by the Food and Drug Administration (FDA) in the United States for the treatment of chronic hepatitis B. Two other brands of alpha interferon approved for hepatitis C treatment have not been formally FDA-approved for hepatitis B.

Pegylated Interferons. The most recent advance in interferon therapy is the development of long-acting (pegylated) interferons that are administered once a week. Currently, there are no published studies of the use of pegylated interferon in the treatment of chronic hepatitis B. Pegylated interferons are fast becoming the standard interferons for the treatment of hepatitis C and undoubtedly will be used for patients with hepatitis B.

Who Should Take Interferon? The U.S. Hepatitis Interventional Therapy (HIT) Study in 1990, the first controlled study of interferon in treating hepatitis B, developed the criteria for selecting patients for treatment. These criteria center on three main issues: how long you've had the disease (chronicity), confirmation of a diagnosis of hepatitis B, and absence of decompensated liver disease. Therefore, patients selected for treatment should have:

- HBsAg positive for at least six months
- positive eAg and HBV DNA
- persistently elevated ALT for at least six months
- compensated liver disease
- liver biopsy compatible with diagnosis of chronic hepatitis B
- no other serious underlying medical condition
- no evidence of hepatic failure (ascites, variceal bleed, encephalopathy)
- bilirubin less than 2 milligrams/deciliter
- albumin greater than 3 grams/deciliter

- prothrombin time less than 3 seconds prolonged beyond control
- platelet count greater than 70,000/microliter
- white blood count greater than 3,000/microliter, polymorphonuclear leucocytes (PMN) greater than 1,500/ microliter
- hematocrit greater than 33 percent

(For a full explanation of technical terms listed above, see Chapter 2.)

Patients should not be pregnant and should have no evidence of other underlying primary liver disease (autoimmune chronic active hepatitis or active alcoholic hepatitis, in particular).

Many patients with chronic hepatitis B may not meet the criteria for treatment. Please note that the above criteria are fairly restrictive and define only a subpopulation of the patients with chronic hepatitis B. For example, in the 1990 HIT trial 545 patients with chronic hepatitis B were screened, but only 169 actually met the criteria and began treatment.

Your doctor may prescribe interferon therapy alone (monotherapy) or interferon in combination with other drugs (combination therapy). In the following sections, I will discuss variations of interferon therapy and how doctors measure response to treatment.

Interferon Monotherapy. The standard regimen of interferon therapy for chronic hepatitis B is five million units (5 MU) given by subcutaneous (under the skin) injection six times a week (usually Monday through Saturday), or 10 MU three times a week (usually Monday, Wednesday, and Friday) for 16 to 32 weeks. Investigators have tried higher doses, daily dosing, and longer courses of interferon with minor improvements in overall response.

Prednisone "Priming" Followed by Interferon. Clinical investigators have found that Prednisone treatment followed by the withdrawal of prednisone stimulates the immune reaction to hepatitis B. On the basis of this observation, some investigators have used prednisone and prednisone withdrawal (priming) prior to interferon to enhance the antiviral effect of interferon.

A subgroup of noncirrhotic patients with low level ALT, less than 100 IU/L (international units per liter), appear to benefit from prednisone pretreatment. The regimen begins with 60 milligrams per day of prednisone, and the dose is decreased every two weeks by 20 milligrams per day with a two-week "washout" (no prednisone) just before starting interferon. Interferon monotherapy is then administered as described above.

However, this approach remains controversial because it is potentially dangerous, especially in cirrhotic patients where the treatment has the potential to precipitate severe hepatitis and liver failure. Prednisone priming is not recommended unless the treating physician is experienced in its use.

Interferon Plus Lamivudine. The combination of interferon with lamivudine [see section below, "What Is Lamivudine (EPIVIR-HBV®)?] is appealing because these two agents have proven individually effective against hepatitis B, and they exert their antiviral effects in completely different ways. Nonetheless, results with current regimens have been disappointing. In these studies researchers administered lamivudine initially to reduce viral load before introducing interferon. The decision to use this sequential treatment was based upon prior studies demonstrating that patients with lower viral loads were more likely to respond to interferon.

One trial of 228 naive patients (people who had not been previously treated) from Europe, Canada, and Australia failed to demonstrate a benefit of combination treatment over either interferon or lamivudine monotherapy. A second trial of 238 nonresponders to interferon failed to demonstrate a benefit of combination treatment over lamivudine monotherapy. We do not know yet whether different treatment protocols, doses, or duration of therapy would improve the effectiveness of combination treatment. Currently, we don't have enough clinical evidence to support a recommendation for routine use of the combination of interferon plus lamivudine in the treatment of chronic hepatitis B.

Interferon Plus Ribavirin. Ribavirin is a nucleoside analogue of guanosine and has antiviral activity against a variety of DNA and RNA viruses. In addition, ribavirin modifies the immune response and enhances the antiviral activity of interferon.

Scientists are still investigating the exact mechanism that causes ribavirin to act against hepatitis B. Ribavirin, when used alone as monotherapy, has no beneficial effect in the treatment of hepatitis B; it is effective only in combination with interferon.

Because ribavirin breaks down red blood cells, patients should have a hemoglobin concentration greater than 12 grams per deciliter (gms/dl) in women and 13 gms/dl in men. Additionally, candidates should:

- have platelet count greater than 100,000 platelets per microliter
- have no active cardiovascular disease
- practice adequate contraception to avoid pregnancy

The breakdown of red blood cells (hemolysis) is a common side effect of ribavirin, necessitating dose reductions in approximately 8 percent of patients. This adverse reaction occurs early in treatment and typically stabilizes after the first four weeks. Rarely does a patient withdraw completely from therapy due to this reaction.

Other side effects that occur more frequently with combination therapy than with interferon monotherapy include shortness of breath, throat irritation, itching, rash, nausea, difficulty sleeping, and loss of appetite. Twenty to 26 percent of patients will require dose reductions related to any of the above side effects.

An uncontrolled pilot study investigated the combination of interferon plus ribavirin in 24 patients with the "pre-core mutation" of hepatitis B (see "Precore Mutation" section below and Chapter 2), who failed a prior course of interferon treatment. Patients received five million units three times a week (5 MU tiw) plus 1.0 to 1.2 grams daily (1.2 g/d) of ribavirin for 12 months. They were followed for an additional 12 months after treatment was discontinued. Many patients were intolerant of treatment, and 21 percent had to stop ribavirin. After treatment and 12 months of follow-up, 50 percent were HBV DNA negative but only 21 percent had normal ALT levels. Although paired biopsies (pre-treatment compared to post-treatment) were available for only a few patients, the biopsies showed improvement in the sustained responders.

This early promising experience awaits confirmation of a properly controlled clinical trial. Until such data are available, widespread use of combination interferon plus ribavirin in treatment of chronic hepatitis cannot be recommended.

Measuring Response to Interferon Treatment. Effective therapy reduces liver cell damage, clears hepatitis B, and blocks the progression of inflammation and fibrosis to cirrhosis. We know if the treatment works by measuring your response in three ways:

- **ALT (SGPT).** Hepatitis B invades liver cells, and your body's immune response attempts to clear the infection by attacking the virus. This response damages the liver cells, and ALT, an enzyme within the liver cell, leaks through the cells' membranes into the bloodstream. Interferon enhances the immune response to hepatitis B. Because a part of the liver injury is due to immune reactions, interferon therapy may initially increase the degree of liver injury and elevate ALT levels (see Figure 8B).

With resolution of the viral infection, the liver injury ceases and ALT levels normalize. Normal ALT levels imply that liver injury has stopped or is diminished. Therefore, ALT levels are commonly used as a measure of effectiveness of treatment ("biochemical response").

- **HBV DNA, eAg.** When you have active hepatitis B infection, your blood contains HBV DNA plus e antigen (usually) or HBV DNA alone (because of pre-core mutation, which blocks the production of e antigen). Effective anti-viral treatment clears HBV DNA and e antigen from the bloodstream. Responders typically clear HBV DNA first; clearance of e antigen follows (see Figure 8B). Clearing the e antigen can also be associated with development of e antibody. This

FIGURE 8B: CLINICAL COURSE IN A PATIENT WHO WAS SUCCESSFULLY TREATED WITH INTERFERON.

ALT (IU/L)

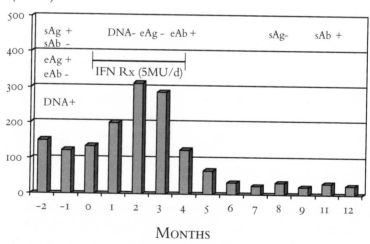

MONTHS

LEGEND 8B: Prior to treatment the patient had biopsy evidence of chronic hepatitis, and the serology demonstrated active viral replication (eAg and DNA positive). ALT was elevated (nl < 40 IU/L) prior to treatment and flared with interferon therapy. The sequence of events during treatment was clearance of DNA, loss of eAg, and development of eAb. After treatment the ALT remained normal, sAg cleared, and the patient developed sAb.

change, commonly called seroconversion, is associated with clinical remission. Clearance of HBV DNA and e antigen and development of e antibody are classified as "virologic or viral responses."

In long-term follow-up, the majority of patients who have undergone seroconversion from e antigen to e antibody ultimately lose hepatitis B surface antigen and many develop hepatitis B surface antibody. Patients with the latter response do not relapse, and they remain in long-term remission.

- **Liver Biopsy.** Liver biopsies define the extent of inflammation in the liver and the amount of fibrosis. Effective therapy is associated with a decrease in inflammation and fibrosis. Improvement in the microscopic appearance of liver biopsies is often called a "histologic (cell and tissue) response."

My last biopsy showed moderate to severe fibrosis. I started interferon and had an immediate flare. My immune system went whammo— which meant it was working. The flare increased, and after eight weeks my blood tests went off the charts. It looked like it was killing me.

The doctors took me off, then put me back on ten days later when the flare happened again. They called me a nonresponder. But a month later, the doctors changed their minds when my e antigen disappeared. Now I was a responder, even though I still had the surface antigen.

Two years later, I got rid of the surface antigen, but I think I still have a small amount of the virus in my liver because I don't have surface antibodies. You really want surface antibodies.

One-third of us respond to interferon like I did. Out of those who respond, about 35 to 70 percent go on to lose the surface antigen. I was real lucky!

Larry

How effective is interferon? Looking at experimental statistics gives us important information, but when you are the person who's taking interferon, you want to know how to measure success or failure. Physicians have a special vocabulary they use to describe a patient's response:

- **Virologic (Viral) Response (The "Gold" Standard).** We define complete viral response as the clearance of HBV DNA and e antigen during or after a course of therapy. Seroconversion to e antibody is associated with more durable viral remission. If the viral response

FIGURE 8C. INTERFERON THERAPY OF CHRONIC HEPATITIS B

% OF PATIENTS WITH SUSTAINED SEROLOGIC CLEARANCE

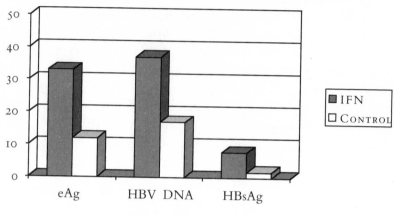

VIRAL MARKERS

LEGEND 8C: These results were from an analysis of 15 randomized controlled trials, representing results in 837 adult patients with chronic hepatitis B (Wong, D.K.H., A.M. Cheung, K. O'Rourke, C.D. Naylor, A.S. Detsky, J. Heathcote. Effect of Alpha-Interferon Treatment in Patients with Hepatitis B e Antigen-Positive Chronic Hepatitis B. A Meta-Analysis. *Annals of Internal Medicine.* 1993; 119:312-323). Sustained remission in the viral infection (persistently negative eAg and HBV DNA), 6 to 12 months after treatment, occurs in 30% to 40% of patients treated with interferon. HBsAg clearance is less frequent, but with years of follow-up the majority of patients who remain eAg and DNA negative will lose HBsAg.

persists for six months after stopping interferon, the patient is classified as a "sustained responder."

One analysis of 16 randomized controlled trials of interferon treatment of naive patients indicated that 33 percent cleared e antigen (compared to 12 percent for untreated controls), and 37 percent cleared HBV DNA (compared to 17 percent for untreated controls) (see Figure 8C).

Sustained responders typically develop e antibody, rarely relapse, and most clear hepatitis B surface antigen in long-term follow-up. "Relapsers" clear HBV DNA and e entigen on treatment but do not develop e antibody. When treatment is discontinued, HBV DNA and e antigen return. "Nonresponders" fail to clear either HBV DNA or e antigen at any time during therapy.

- **Biochemical Response.** During interferon therapy, a responder will typically exhibit a flare in ALT with elevations two to threefold or more above pretreatment levels. The elevation in ALT usually occurs after six to ten weeks of treatment during viral clearance when levels of HBV DNA are declining and e antigen is disappearing. After viral eradication, inflammation and injury cease and ALT decreases to the normal range. Seroconversion from e antigen to e antibody is usually associated with normal ALT levels.
- **Histologic (Cell and Tissue) Response.** A sustained viral response to interferon therapy is associated with improvement in the condition of the liver cells and tissue. Improvement observed during microscopic examination of liver biopsies is due mostly to reduced inflammatory activity. In the long term, successful interferon therapy may inhibit, or possibly reverse, liver fibrosis.

Predictors of Response. Certain factors may correlate with a better chance to clear hepatitis B with interferon. Of all the following factors, the most important is a low level of HBV DNA:

- low levels of HBV DNA, less than 200 picograms per milliliter
- shorter duration of infection
- female gender
- absence of HIV
- ALT levels greater than 100 IU/L (international units per liter)

The Patient's Experience: Interferon Injections. Most patients are nervous about interferon injections and concerned about dealing with medications and the side effects of treatment. In my experience, patients quickly learn how to give themselves injections. Most people think of the deep muscle injections they get for flu shots, and they panic about doing this to themselves. Interferon injections are much easier to administer because they are subcutaneous. Subcutaneous means you have to get the needle only under the skin and not deep into muscle.

I was really nervous about learning how to give myself a shot. When I came into the office, the nurse was looking all around for an orange to practice on. She never did find it. So we used the pad on the exam table, then a tissue box. It was funny, and it made me laugh—something I never expected to happen.

The first couple of times I did it myself at home, I put the needle in too horizontally. I was going push, push, push and nothing happened. I got awful bruises.

Back to the nurse. She told me to pinch my skin between two fingers, hold the syringe like a dart and go in straight at a 90° angle. That worked!

Marla

It's important that you ask questions and practice injections under a nurse's supervision until you feel comfortable. You should be taught about storing and preparing the drug for injection, sterile technique, how to pick injection sites, and how to dispose of needles. Be sure to ask for the helpful teaching material and videotapes that pharmaceutical companies give to physicians for their patients' use.

I recommend that the first shot be given in the office. Although it's highly unlikely for a patient to have an immediate adverse reaction, we observe the patient for a couple of hours.

Interferon Side Effects. Each person reacts differently to interferon. The most common complaints are flu-like symptoms because when you get an actual case of the flu, your body fights back by sending interferon to attack the invader. Interferon is at least partially responsible for tired, achy, and feverish symptoms.

I was on interferon for ten months. It didn't bother me. Only two things bothered me. The first night was hell. Then later on, the interferon had an adverse effect on my blood count, and I was next to collapsing. I couldn't even walk up the stairs.

They gave me two units of blood and dropped my dosage from five to three million. I wasn't getting better or worse, just maintaining.

Howard

Some people don't have many symptoms during interferon treatment; others suffer from chills, muscle aches, nausea, even diarrhea. These symptoms usually subside after the first few weeks. Weight loss is also a common side effect, but it tends to persist throughout the course of therapy. Some patients are able to maintain their weight and improve their energy by using supplements, such as Ensure Plus®, Resource®, and Suplena®.

To help with side effects, I recommend two regular strength tablets of acetaminophen (Tylenol®), ibuprofen, or naproxen, just before you take the injection. The latter two drugs can irritate your stomach and should not be taken frequently. Medications that are safer for your stomach but similarly effective include celecoxib (Celebrex®) and rofecoxib (Vioxx®). Side effects may also be reduced if you're well hydrated before and after the injection (two glasses before an injection and about two-and-a-half quarts of fluid a day).

For fatigue, it may help to have a daily nap or rest period. Paradoxically, some patients feel their fatigue is relieved by daily activity, including exercise. Eat small, more frequent meals if you're losing your appetite. To avoid skin reactions, rotate the injection sites.

During interferon therapy you will need frequent blood tests. The main reason for doing these blood tests is to be certain your blood counts are adequate. Interferon reduces the white blood cell count and the platelet count. This effect of interferon is directly related to the dose used; higher doses cause a greater lowering of the counts. Sometimes the dose of interferon may need to be reduced or even discontinued.

Particularly distressing side effects that occur in a minority of patients include depression, mental changes, and hair loss. Depression on interferon usually occurs in patients with a pre-treatment history of depression. However, it can occur in any patient, bears close supervision, and may require reducing the dosage or even stopping treatment. In some cases, in order to continue interferon, your physician may prescribe medication to control symptoms of depression (Zoloft®, Elavil®, Effexor®, or Prozac®). If hair is lost during treatment, it usually grows back after treatment stops. Your physician will monitor you closely to watch out for other rare side effects, including thyroid disease or the development of other autoimmune disorders (see Chapter 4).

Be sure to tell your doctor if any of these symptoms appear:

- thoughts of suicide
- thoughts of homicide
- sustained fever (greater than 102° F) or other signs of infection
- generalized rash
- any symptoms that are interfering with your daily activity

Interferon may affect your ability to fight infection. Do not undergo procedures, such as excessive dental work, without checking with your doctor first; your physician may decide to prescribe an antibiotic to protect you.

Generally, most people adjust well. I tell patients to keep busy, exercise, drink lots of water, rest when they need to, socialize. Focus on positive things. Above all, don't let interferon isolate you.

Treatment Tips from Patients. Here are some tips from hepatitis patients who've gone through interferon treatment. Remember, what works for one person may not work for you. Once you become familiar with these drugs, you'll find your own comfort level.

> *For me, drinking lots of water helped. If I didn't stay hydrated, I felt worse.*

> *I lost some hair. The good news is that my hair came back thicker, which, believe me, I could use. All in all, hair loss was a small price to pay for the reward of clearing the virus.*

> *Massage helped me manage the aches and pains. I had to find the money for it, but sometimes you just have to admit that you're going through a hard time—and you need to be extra good to yourself.*

> *Interferon treatment reduced my stamina. I felt weak, but I did not get depressed. I was scared at first, but my husband was very supportive. I got thyroid problems from the interferon, but it worked for me.*

> *I dropped 20 pounds because I had no appetite—and I'm pretty thin as it is. My stomach was ... I don't know, I just couldn't seem to eat. You really have to make sure you eat, even if you have to take several smaller meals throughout the day.*

> *The people in my support group decided the two major things that helped were to get a lot of rest and to have a positive attitude. What's really interesting is that in spite of the side effects, no one was sorry they had tried interferon.*

> *I'm a fair bit more irritable. So I apologize and say I'm not feeling well. It's me, not you. I do a fair amount of apologizing.*

It's a peculiar kind of headache. I call it the interferon headache. Also, it seems as though I'm more forgetful. Now I write everything—and I mean everything—down!

In the morning and at night, I feel nauseous. If I eat, the nausea goes away. I have to concentrate on eating. And if I eat right before or after an injection, I don't have side effects.

For me, the fatigue is the tough part. I got over the slight fever and upset stomach in the first couple of days. But I do get tired, and I just have to rest more. About midway through the treatment, I had to go on an antidepressant, and that's helped me a lot.

I've had to learn to say no. It's amazing how you can simplify your work life if you have no choice. And I've learned not to schedule too many appointments in one day. If I'm running from one thing to another, I'm wiped out at the end of the day.

Lamivudine

I started interferon in March of 1990. It was the first time I heard of interferon. There were lots of side effects, especially depression. I was given the impression it was all in my head. "Keep at it," the nurse said. I was throwing up a lot—every day for six months, and I was especially sick after injections.

I think it did me more harm than good. I went from fibrosis to cirrhosis. I was in bad shape before the interferon and worse shape after it. In 1991, transplants for hepatitis B were not done. My only alternative was to accept death.

I was told I had three years, but I made it to 1995 when tests showed my liver was decompensating. I went on the transplant list and simultaneously was initiated on lamivudine on a study. I begged my doctor for lamivudine, and I got it on a compassionate use basis. Within 30 days, my viral replication went down to one percent and now it's less than that.

Stan

What Is Lamivudine (EPIVIR-HBV®)? Lamivudine is a nucleoside analogue in pill form. It is FDA-approved for hepatitis B as EPIVIR-

HBV®. Lamivudine binds to certain genes of the virus that allow the virus to jump from DNA to RNA and back to DNA. This activity is called reverse transcriptase and is a property not only of hepatitis B but also of the human immunodeficiency virus (HIV). In simple terms, lamivudine blocks the life cycle of the virus, and the virus fails to reproduce.

The drug was initially developed for use in HIV-positive patients. However, when lamivudine was given to patients co-infected with both HIV and HBV, it acted against hepatitis B as well. A small pilot study of 32 patients showed lamivudine was effective against hepatitis B and defined the optimum dose as 100 milligrams daily. This initial experience led to larger clinical trials that defined the effectiveness of the drug.

> *I was on interferon from March until May. It was bad stuff. Then the doctor called and said to stop taking it; it was not helping me. I was so thankful I didn't have to take that stuff anymore. With EPIVIR®, I have no side effects. Last year I had a transplant, and I still take EPIVIR®.*
>
> Cindy

Who Should Take Lamivudine? The current accepted criteria for selecting patients for treatment were developed in the initial controlled studies of lamivudine in the United States and Asia. The criteria are similar to those used for interferon (see above section, Who Should Take Interferon?), except for three differences:

- bilirubin less than 2.5 milligrams per deciliter
- albumin greater than 3.5 grams per deciliter
- platelet count greater than 100,000 per cubic millimeter

Although lamivudine is FDA-approved for treatment of noncirrhotic or compensated chronic hepatitis B, many investigators are using the drug to clear hepatitis B in patients with more advanced liver disease. An increasing number of reports indicate that lamivudine is tolerated by cirrhotic patients, even those with decompensated liver disease who are awaiting transplantation.

> *I've got cirrhosis. The doctors put me on EPIVIR®. Originally, they told me it would only be for six months. After six months, my jaundice finally went away, and I got to a point where we weren't sure if I had*

hepatitis or not. I was positive for antigens but my DNA was negative. My doctor said if it were his body, he'd stay on EPIVIR®. In April I got approved to be on the list for a liver transplant.

Al

In 1997, I was coming back from a bus trip, and I didn't feel well. I thought, "Gee, this has been a long trip with lots of meetings, and I'm just tired." I lay on the couch at home. It felt like I had the flu. I woke up, was sick to my stomach—and vomited blood everywhere. I wasn't conscious by the time I got to the hospital. The doctors told me I needed a liver transplant.

EPIVIR®, also called 3TC, was being used as an antiviral for HIV then, and they were testing it for people with hepatitis B. Two months after starting EPIVIR®, I went antigen negative, but a year later I had a breakthrough.

I'm still taking it, though. The doctors discussed it and said EPIVIR® was treating some portion of the hepatitis. They decided to leave me on it and see if it did some good. I don't have flare-ups any longer.

Roberta

In November of 1998, I was in the hospital for ascites. I also had bleeding problems. The floor they put me on was like going in for last rites. I never saw so many dying, diseased patients.

The doctor told my children I had only two weeks left to live, and they should say their goodbyes because I would become mentally confused. The doctors drained most of the fluid, and I went home.

That December, I got a second opinion and enrolled in a trial, a study of lamivudine. I've been on lamivudine ever since—150 milligrams a day. I don't have ascites or bleeding problems anymore. And it's been two years!

Richard

Patients should not be pregnant or show any evidence of other underlying primary liver disease (autoimmune chronic active hepatitis or active alcoholic hepatitis, in particular).

What doses of lamivudine are used? The preferred and standard regimen for use of lamivudine as initial therapy for chronic hepatitis B is 100 milligrams daily for 52 weeks. Lower doses suppress HBV DNA levels but do not make them undetectable. Higher doses are not necessary to inhibit reproduction of the virus.

Measuring Response to Lamivudine Treatment. As with interferon therapy, we measure the effectiveness of treatment by normalization of ALT levels, clearance of HBV DNA and e antigen, and reduction in inflammation and fibrosis on liver biopsy. Unlike interferon, lamivudine does not stimulate an immune reaction to hepatitis B but primarily inhibits viral replication. Therefore, lamivudine is not associated with an increase in ALT during viral clearance that occurs early in treatment. Normal ALT levels parallel the clearing of HBV DNA and e antigen.

With lamivudine treatment, HBV DNA and e antigen typically clear from the bloodstream within four to eight weeks (see Figure 8D). Approximately 20 percent of patients will undergo seroconversion from e antigen to e antibody. In long-term follow-up, many patients who

FIGURE 8D: COURSE OF A PATIENT WHO WAS TREATED WITH LAMIVUDINE.

ALT (IU/L)

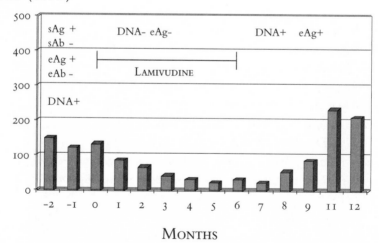

MONTHS

LEGEND 8D: Prior to treatment the patient had active viral replication as demonstrated by positive eAg and HBV DNA in blood. Treatment with lamivudine effectively suppressed viral replication, and eAg and HBV DNA became negative. However, once treatment stopped, viral replication resumed, and both eAg and HBV DNA became positive.

undergo seroconversion from e antigen to e antibody remain in long-term remission; the virus does not recur in their blood. Serial liver biopsies show a reduction in inflammation.

How effective is lamivudine? We classify the response to lamivudine in a similar way as interferon (see above section, Measuring Response to Interferon Treatment).

*   **Virologic (Viral) Response (The "Gold" Standard).** Complete viral response is defined as clearance of HBV DNA and e antigen during or after a course of therapy. If you clear e antigen and HBV DNA for six months after stopping lamivudine, you are called a "sustained responder." If you also convert to e antibody, your response is associated with a long-term sustained viral remission.

    In the U.S. multi-center trial, 66 patients were treated with lamivudine (100 milligrams daily for 52 weeks) and compared to 71 controls receiving a placebo. Follow-up extended for 16 weeks beyond the end of treatment. All patients in this trial were positive for e antigen and had abnormal ALT (see Figure 8E).

FIGURE 8E: RESPONSE TO LAMIVUDINE (100 mg/d) IN THE U.S. TRIAL.

% OF PATIENTS WITH ON-TREATMENT RESPONSE

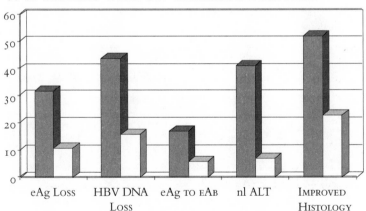

MARKERS OF RESPONSE

LEGEND 8E: The percentage of patients who were responding to lamivudine at week 52 of treatment are shown. About 30% to 40% demonstrated clearance of eAg and/or HBV DNA. Only 17% underwent eAg to eAb seroconversion, but more than 40% normalized ALT and more than 50% had improvement in liver disease on liver biopsy.

Patients treated with lamivudine were more likely to clear HBV DNA, lose e antigen, develop e antibody, normalize ALT, and improve histology on liver biopsy. HBV DNA tended to return, but e antigen remained negative during the 16 weeks of follow-up. In comparison with other studies, the rate of return of HBV DNA after 12 months of treatment is less than that seen with either three-month or six-month courses. In addition, lamivudine is well tolerated and has few, if any, side effects.

In the Asian study, 143 patients were treated with lamivudine (100 milligrams daily for 52 weeks) and compared to 73 patients receiving a placebo. The durability of response could not be assessed because there was no follow-up period after discontinuing the drug. (Figure 8F shows the results.) As in the U.S. trial, patients treated with lamivudine were more likely to improve liver histology, lose HBV DNA, and become negative for e antigen. Also, lamivudine was well tolerated, and patients experienced few side effects.

FIGURE 8F: RESPONSE TO LAMIVUDINE (100 mg/d) IN THE ASIAN TRIAL.

% OF PATIENTS WITH ON-TREATMENT RESPONSE

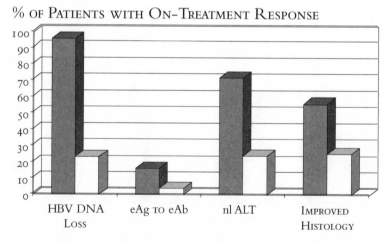

MARKERS OF RESPONSE

LEGEND 8F: The percentage of patients with response to lamivudine after 52 weeks of treatment is shown: 96% cleared HBV DNA at some time during the course of treatment. Seroconversion from eAg to eAb occurred in 16%. More than 70% normalized ALT, and more than 50% had improvement in liver disease on liver biopsy.

In summary, lamivudine is highly effective at suppressing hepatitis B, but after treatment is stopped, relapse is common. Fifteen to 20 percent of treated patients, however, may undergo seroconversion from e antigen to e antibody and enjoy long-term remission from active infection.

- **Biochemical Response.** During lamivudine therapy, a responder typically normalizes or markedly reduces ALT levels. A flare of ALT on treatment does not occur unless there is a breakthrough in viral replication or the development of the YMDD mutation.

  When treatment is stopped, there is danger of a major flare or increase in ALT associated with significant liver injury. Patients with cirrhosis and compromised hepatic reserve are at risk for decompensation and development of liver failure during such a flare. For this reason, patients with cirrhosis who are treated with lamivudine should stop treatment only under close medical supervision. Seroconversion from e antigen to e antibody often results in normal ALT levels.

- **Histologic (Cell and Tissue) Response.** Sustained viral response to lamivudine therapy is associated with improvement in the condition of liver cells and tissue. This improvement, observed during microscopic examination of liver biopsies, results mostly from reduced inflammatory activity. In the long term, successful lamivudine therapy may inhibit or possibly reverse liver fibrosis.

Predictors of Response. Unlike interferon therapy, nearly all patients respond to lamivudine with suppression of HBV DNA and e antigen. This response is similar regardless of ALT, HBV DNA level, liver biopsy findings, age, race, weight, or the presence of cirrhosis.

Precore Mutation. A unique circumstance occurs when HBV DNA is positive but e antigen is negative. This phenomenon is due to a spontaneously occurring mutation in the genes of hepatitis B near (pre-core) the gene coding for the core antigen. The mutation occurs in the region of the e antigen gene and prevents expression of e antigen. Thus, patients with this mutation (pre-core mutation) have active viral replication, as defined by positive HBV DNA, but lack e antigen.

Some investigators have suggested that patients with this mutation are more likely to experience aggressive disease and that they are more resistant to treatment. In contrast, recent evidence suggests that these patients may respond to either interferon or lamivudine.

YMDD Mutations. YMDD mutations of hepatitis B occur mostly, but not exclusively, in patients taking lamivudine. The mutation allows the virus to escape from lamivudine. The result is that blood which was previously negative tests positive for HBV DNA. The YMDD mutations are alterations in the genes of hepatitis B. These mutations render the virus resistant to lamivudine. Therefore, in the presence of lamivudine, YMDD mutations of hepatitis B replicate.

Lamivudine targets the gene coding for the DNA polymerase of the hepatitis B genome. The normal sequence of nucleotides of the DNA polymerase encodes for the four amino acids: Y (tyrosine), M (methionine), D (aspartate), and D (aspartate). So, although the lamivudine resistant mutants are called YMDD mutants, in fact YMDD refers to the naturally occurring ("wild type") DNA polymerase.

There are two common mutations of YMDD, YIDD (I=isoleucine) and YVDD (V=valine). These mutations distort the binding regions within the DNA polymerase gene and make lamivudine ineffective in blocking viral replication. In simple terms, mutations of YMDD block lamivudine effects on hepatitis B. The result is the re-emergence of infection in a patient who was previously responding. HBV DNA, despite initial suppression, then becomes positive during lamivudine treatment.

> *After three years on lamivudine and famciclovir, my hepatitis B virus started mutating. My DNA viral load went up drastically in three months—from 2,200 to 261,000. "Hey," I said, "I'm a mutant!"*
>
> *About six months later, my counts went down. My doctor hasn't a clue and says he has never seen anything like it. The effect of the mutation, if it did take place, might have been masked. But I am not going to take tests to determine which mutant I have, if any, until the HBV DNA starts going up again. And I hope that doesn't happen.*
>
> *Doug*

In the U.S. trial, 32 percent of patients treated with lamivudine for one year developed YMDD mutations. Other studies show that up to 50 percent of patients treated for three years developed the YMDD mutation.

Patients with YMDD mutations on treatment can experience hepatitis-like or flu-like symptoms, and their ALT levels typically increase. If hepatitis occurs, it is usually mild and self-limited as long as lamivudine is continued. The patient remains positive for HBV DNA, but the ALT usually regresses back to the normal range. Severe hepatitis has occurred during the emergence of YMDD mutation if lamivudine is discontinued. For this reason, doctors currently recommend that lamivudine be continued despite the emergence of this resistant strain of virus.

Side Effects. Lamivudine, in the doses used to treat hepatitis B, is surprisingly free of side effects. Molecules related to lamivudine have been reported to cause injury to liver cells, resulting in acidosis and even liver failure. However, none of these reactions have occurred with the doses of lamivudine used in therapy of patients with chronic hepatitis B.

Thymosin-alpha1 (Zadaxin®)

Thymosin-alpha1 has been investigated in three clinical trials of the treatment of hepatitis B. The initial uncontrolled trial indicated that thymosin treatment might be equivalent or superior to interferon and have fewer side effects. However, two randomized controlled trials of thymosin for chronic hepatitis B gave conflicting results. Thymosin is not currently FDA-approved, but additional clinical trials are underway. For this reason, most clinicians have not considered thymosin in the arsenal of treatment options for chronic hepatitis B.

Famciclovir (Famvir ®) and Ganciclovir (Cytovene®)

Famciclovir, like lamivudine, is a nucleoside analogue that acts against hepatitis B. Studies of patients infected with hepatitis B demonstrate that famiciclovir inhibits HBV DNA—but to a lesser extent than lamivudine. In addition, famciclovir is ineffective against YMDD mutations that are resistant to lamivudine. Therefore, famciclovir is limited to treatment of hepatitis B patients who are intolerant of lamivudine. Some doctors use the combination of lamivudine and famciclovir.

> *Four years ago, an absolutely routine physical showed there was something wrong with my liver functions. I had chronic active hepatitis B. Within six months my legs and belly were swollen. My doctor washed his hands of me and told me I had two months to live, and there was nothing left to do.*
>
> *I was mad as hell. I did a search and read, read, read about hepatitis B. I found my own way. I called a doctor at New York University, and asked him to give me the lamivudine/famciclovir combination.*

He was proud of me. Over the next six months, I went undetectable.

Zach

Ganciclovir is related to famciclovir and also shows activity against hepatitis B. However, the drug is poorly absorbed in pill form and must be given intravenously. The effectiveness of a well-absorbed form of ganciclovir (Valtrex®) against hepatitis B is unknown. Currently, both famciclovir and ganciclovir appear to have a limited role in the treatment of hepatitis B.

Side Effects. Famciclovir and ganciclovir are well tolerated with few side effects. At high doses patients may develop bone marrow suppression with both low white cell count and low platelet count.

I have religiously followed my anti-viral regimen of lamivudine and famciclovir for three years. I have no side effects at all. If anything, my health is better. I used to get leg cramps and skin rashes, and now I don't get them anymore.

Julius

Adefovir Dipivoxil

What Is Adefovir? Adefovir is also a nucleoside analogue, similar but distinct from lamivudine. A pill, typically taken in doses ranging from 5 to 30 milligrams a day, adefovir acts against a number of viruses, including hepatitis B, retroviruses, and herpes viruses. It markedly inhibits both wild type and YMDD mutations of hepatitis B and is effective against both lamivudine-resistant and famciclovir-resistant strains of HBV. In simple terms, adefovir blocks the life cycle of the virus, and the virus fails to reproduce.

I've had chronic hepatitis B for almost five years. I was infected via sexual transmission. Now, of course, I'm a strong advocate of safe sex!
I've been on adefovir twice—Phase I and Phase II studies. Both times my HBV DNA dropped to nil but flared after treatment stopped. I didn't have any side effects the entire time I was on the drug, and my liver enzymes were high normal.

Although long-term side effects are not yet known, I would definitely consider taking this drug on a long-term basis to suppress the virus until a cure is found.

Betty

Adefovir was shown to be effective against hepatitis B in a phase II study where 20 percent of treated patients developed e antigen seroconversion after only 12 weeks of treatment. Like lamivudine, adefovir dipivoxil suppresses viral replication but fails to eliminate the virus in the majority of cases. However, it is effective against not only wild-type but also YMDD mutations of hepatitis B.

Who Should Take Adefovir? At the time of this writing, adefovir dipivoxil was not yet FDA-approved for treatment of hepatitis B. It is currently available only through clinical trials or compassionate use protocols. I anticipate that it will be recommended primarily for treatment of patients who develop YMDD mutation during treatment with lamivudine. Most likely, adefovir will be given in conjunction with lamivudine and may also be effective as a single agent. Researchers are still studying the long-term safety, effectiveness, and therapeutic role of adefovir at this time.

Measuring Response. The effectiveness of adefovir is determined by measuring changes in ALT, HBV DNA, and liver histology (see the Measuring Response/Lamivudine section).

Side Effects. A recent publication indicated that adefovir also might be highly effective, even in low doses, after liver transplantation. However, one concern with the drug has been potential renal (kidney) toxicity. Adefovir causes renal dysfunction and has been associated with low phosphate, usually when given in doses of 60 to 120 milligrams a day.

Doctors can reduce the side effects by lowering the dose or stopping treatment. Adefovir inhibits hepatitis B at doses ranging from 5 to 30 milligrams a day. However, the transplant drugs used to prevent rejection (cyclosporine, tacrolimus) also impair renal function and may add to the renal toxicity of adefovir. For this reason, most of the cases of post-transplant hepatitis B that have been treated used 5 to 10 milligrams a day of adefovir.

After Treatment, What Next?

When you finish the course of treatment your doctor prescribes, you'll know if you're a nonresponder or a responder. Complete responders maintain a normal ALT and clear HBV DNA on treatment. Sustained responders maintain their complete response after treatment is discontinued. Nonresponders, including partial responders, fail to sustain a normal ALT or clear HBV DNA. What your doctor recommends next depends on your initial response to treatment.

If You Are a Nonresponder to Interferon Monotherapy. For nonresponders, the first question is whether you took the interferon as prescribed. Did you miss doses? If so, why? Were the side effects intolerable? Were you able to take the full dose or was the dosage reduced? If the dosage was reduced, why? The answers to these questions tell the physician how to proceed.

If you missed doses and never received a full course of treatment, one recommendation might be to consider a full standard course of interferon. Some patients experience intolerable side effects, and they can't comply with treatment. When that's the case, simply retreating at the same dose isn't a likely option unless other treatment can minimize side effects. For example, if the dosage was reduced or stopped due to depression, it may be possible to retreat with interferon after treating the depression. If the dose was reduced because of severe lowering of white blood cells or platelets, you may be able to tolerate retreatment with interferon by also taking drugs to increase white cells (Neupogen®) or red cells (Epogen®).

Doctors must address these and other issues because current protocols involving retreatment usually use higher doses and longer duration interferon, or the combination of interferon plus ribavirin. Obviously, patients intolerant to interferon therapy are not likely to tolerate these retreatment protocols.

The other main option for retreatment is lamivudine. Nearly all patients who have failed interferon treatment can then take lamivudine and suppress HBV DNA. The concern regarding retreatment is that most patients (except those who convert from e antigen to e antibody) may then be committed to life-long treatment—and long-term lamivudine treatment is associated with the high likelihood of the emergence of YMDD mutations that are lamivudine-resistant.

If You Are a Nonresponder to Lamivudine. This is rare. Nearly all treated patients suppress hepatitis B on treatment. However, one option for nonresponders to prior courses of lamivudine is to consider interferon or a trial of famciclovir. Another option is to consider long-term suppressive treatment with lamivudine. Currently, there are few options for patients with the YMDD mutation; the only promising therapy, adefovir dipivoxil, is not yet FDA-approved.

If You Are a Responder. A sustained response is the most desirable outcome. That is, you clear the hepatitis B virus on treatment (normal ALT and negative DNA), and you sustain the complete response even after treatment is withdrawn. Most patients with a sustained response have cleared the virus from their blood and have improved their liver biopsy (fewer inflammatory cells and less damage).

Long-term sustained responders (more than three years) may have halted the progression of their liver disease and may have actually cleared hepatitis B completely. However, there is always the risk that hepatitis B may only be dormant and reactivate, flaring at a later date. Patients should continue to undergo periodic blood tests and physical examinations.

Continuing Care. People with hepatitis B are at risk for progressive liver injury, cirrhosis, complications of end-stage disease, and may ultimately require liver transplantation for survival. Additionally, these patients are at risk for developing liver cancer (hepatoma). Thus, general medical advice includes ongoing physical examinations by a physician and blood tests of liver function. Cirrhotic patients with hepatitis B may need periodic measurement of alpha-fetoprotein and ultrasound examinations to detect early liver cancer (see Chapter 10).

You should understand that the combination of alcohol and hepatitis B can cause early progression to cirrhosis and liver failure. Active alcoholism is a contraindication to liver transplantation.

Hepatitis B Vaccine

Once you have chronic hepatitis B, the hepatitis B vaccine will not protect you, but it will protect your loved ones. The vaccine grants them immunity and shields them from infection.

History. In 1969, Baruch Blumberg, M.D., Ph.D. (who discovered the antigen that detected hepatitis B in blood), Irving Millman, Ph.D., and colleagues developed the hepatitis B vaccine from partially purified hepatitis B surface antigen that was extracted from the blood of asymptomatic carriers. Millions of people received protection from this form of the vaccine, and it is still used in some countries, such as China and Korea.

Soon after this vaccine became widely available in 1982, laboratories in the United States and Europe created recombinant forms of the vaccine. Maurice Hilleman, Ph.D., led the team that produced the surface antigen in yeast cells, the method we use in the United States today.

The hepatitis B vaccine is the only vaccine that prevents a cancer: hepatocellular carcinoma, cancer of the liver. In the mid-1970s R. Palmer Beasley, M.D., noticed high rates of both hepatitis B and liver cancer in Taiwan and suspected a link. Eventually, he proved that hepatitis B is a major cause of liver cancer. He also showed that 40 percent of hepatitis B worldwide is spread from mother to infants during childbirth and that immunizing newborns prevents 95 percent of these cases.

"These perfectly health(y)-appearing carrier mothers—on their way, however, to chronic liver disease—infected the babies, and the babies almost always became carriers if they were infected by their mothers," said Dr. Beasley.[1] He and his colleagues began a nationwide immunization campaign. The virus carrier rate in Taiwanese children dropped from about 12 percent to 1 percent. Liver cancer rates also dropped.

In theory, we could eventually eradicate hepatitis B with a global vaccination campaign aimed especially at infants. Today, extensive vaccination programs in areas of the world where hepatitis B is highly prevalent, such as China, show great promise. Poverty and politically unstable governments, however, often sidetrack immunization efforts.

> **Resource**: In the U.S., each state has its own immunization regulations. For a chart of state mandates for hepatitis B prevention and implementation, contact the Immunization Action Coalition (IAC) at 651-647-9009. Website: www.immunize.org/laws/hepb.htm

What Is the Hepatitis B Vaccine? The current purified vaccines, Engerix-B® and Recombivax HB®, are made by recombinant DNA technology, which produces pure proteins. There is no risk of inadvertent contamination with hepatitis B or other viruses, such as HIV.

The vaccine is given in a series of three injections, usually at 0, 1, and 6 months for adults and adolescents (see Chapter 12 for children's dosage schedule). Hemodialysis patients, HIV patients, or patients on immunosuppressive drugs may need higher doses. More than 85 percent of children and adolescents and more than 90 to 95 percent of young, healthy adults respond and develop long-lasting immunity from hepatitis B infection.

The combination of hepatitis B vaccine with hepatitis B immune globulin given to newborns of mothers with chronic hepatitis B eliminates risk of infection in 90 to 95 percent of newborns. Long-term follow-up of vaccine recipients indicates that this practice reduces rates of cirrhosis due to hepatitis B and reduces risk of death from either liver failure or liver cancer.

As you can see, most people respond to the vaccination by developing protective antibodies. It is a good idea, however, to ask your doctor to check your antibody response with a simple blood test.

> *I'm a chronic carrier. That means I test positive, but the hepatitis B DNA is undetectable. I haven't done treatment, but my liver biopsy looked really bad. The fact that the DNA is undetectable doesn't mean it didn't do damage.*
>
> *Of course, my husband got vaccinated, but lately he's felt tired, rundown. I said, "Make sure you still have antibodies. Ask the doctor to do a blood test." I was so worried he had hepatitis B.*
>
> *He was okay, but sure enough, his levels had dropped below the minimum. If I hadn't insisted on getting him tested, we wouldn't have known he needed a booster shot.*
>
> *Tracey*

Who Should Be Vaccinated? The Advisory Committee on Immunization Practices (ACIP) recommends the hepatitis B vaccine for all children and adolescents up to the age of 18 and for adults over 18 who are at risk for infection. The vaccine has been recommended as a routine infant vaccination since 1991 and as a routine adolescent vaccination since 1995. If you have hepatitis B, be sure to have all of your sex partners and close personal and household contacts vaccinated.

According to the Centers for Disease Control and Prevention (CDC), you should not get the vaccine if you have had a life-threatening allergic reaction to baker's yeast (used for making bread) or to a previous dose of hepatitis B vaccine. Also, if you are moderately or severely ill, you should wait until you've recovered before getting the vaccine. If in doubt, check with your doctor.

Resource: If you can't afford vaccination shots or don't know where to get them, contact your city, county, or state health department, or call the CDC's Immunization Information Hotline at 1-800-232-2522 (for Spanish language inquiries, call 1-800-232-0233).

Is the Hepatitis B Vaccine Safe? More than 20 million people in the United States and more than 500 million people in the world have been vaccinated. Reported common side effects may include pain at the injection site and a mild to moderate fever. Serious side effects, such as an allergic reaction, are extremely rare. Several federal agencies continually monitor vaccine safety.

There is no confirmed scientific evidence that the vaccine causes chronic illnesses, such as multiple sclerosis, chronic fatigue syndrome, rheumatoid arthritis, or autoimmune disorders. In fact, two studies in the February 1, 2001 issue of *The New England Journal of Medicine* conclude that (1) no association between the hepatitis B vaccination and the development of multiple sclerosis is indicated, and (2) vaccination does not appear to increase the short-term risk of relapse in patients with multiple sclerosis.

Resource: The CDC has issued an interim Vaccine Information Statement (VIS) for hepatitis B vaccine on its Website: www.cdc.gov/nip/publications/vis/vis-hep-b.pdf or on the IAC website: www.immunize.org/vis/hepb00.pdf

Resource: For more information about the hepatitis B vaccine, contact the CDC's Hepatitis Information Line at 1-888-4HEP-CDC (1-888-443-7232), the CDC's Immunization Information Hotline at 1-800-232-2522 (for Spanish language inquiries, call 1-800-232-0233), or call your local or state health department.

Hepatitis A Vaccine

The 1997 National Institutes of Health (NIH) guidelines indicate that hepatitis B patients should get vaccinated for hepatitis A if they don't have detectable antibodies against hepatitis A and therefore are not currently immune. An attack of hepatitis A puts you at increased risk if you already have chronic liver disease.

The vaccine is given in two doses; the first injection is followed by a second injection six months to a year later. The hepatitis A vaccine is not recommended for children under two years of age.

Hepatitis B Immune Globulin (HBIG)

HBIG contains antibodies against the hepatitis B virus. It is primarily given in three situations:

1. to infants born of mothers with hepatitis B
2. to close contacts of patients with chronic hepatitis B
3. to liver recipients with hepatitis B to prevent infection of the transplanted liver

In most cases, the hepatitis B vaccine is given at the same time as HBIG to stimulate immunity against the virus and promote long-term antibody formation. HBIG injections are painful because they are given intramuscularly in relatively large volumes.

> *I get HBIG shots once a month. It's kind of painful because the stuff is pretty thick. They use a full syringe on each side of the hip—$1,000 for each injection!*
>
> *I'm used to it now so I think my body has adjusted. When they use a smaller needle and put the meds in slower, it's better. Everything is getting better all the time since my transplant.*
>
> *Phil*

> *Since my transplant, I take HBIG shots once a month. A lot of men holler when they get those HBIG shots. It hurts. When I come, the nurses say, "Here comes the good patient." I say compared to what I've been through, this is nothing!*
>
> *Henry*

In summary, you have treatment and retreatment options. Work with your doctor to develop a plan. Keep up with research. Scientists are creating more and more effective medications to fight hepatitis B.

Resource: Contact the Hepatitis B Foundation for its updated "HBF Drug Watch: Compounds in Development for Chronic Hepatitis B," 700 East Butler Ave., Doylestown, PA 18901-2697. Phone: 215-489-4900. Email: info@hepb.org. Website: www.hepb.org.

A drug is a substance which when injected into a guinea pig produces a scientific paper.

Anonymous

Reference

[1] Michael A. Snyder, "Research Yields Major Advances in Eradication of HBV–R. Palmer Beasley, M.D.: Resesarcher and Humanitarian," *Hepatitis*. September/October 2000:19.

9

LIVER TRANSPLANTS
A Miracle of Modern Medicine

I got blindsided by this disease in 1995. It snuck up on me. I was feeling weak and tired and couldn't figure out what was going on. I was out on the golf course when all of a sudden I just packed it up.

My doctor ran blood tests and told me it was hepatitis B. He could have told me anything, because I had no idea what he was talking about. I associated it with hepatitis A. He never educated me about what I was really dealing with, nor did he send me to a specialist.

I was jaundiced and felt like I had the flu. Toward the end of four months, the edema came on. By fall, it went away so I forgot about it. I thought it was a passing thing.

Two years later, I was on vacation, and I started feeling bad. My AST and ALT levels were inching up. The doctor walked in the office with X-rays in his hand. "I'm sorry," he said, "really, really sorry. You probably have three years on that liver."

Tom

SOME PEOPLE WITH hepatitis B develop cirrhosis, liver failure, and need a liver transplant to survive. Liver transplantation is the most complicated therapy for people with end-stage hepatitis B, but it currently produces excellent results. In past years, patients who underwent transplantation for hepatitis B had high rates of recurring disease, poor graft function, and reduced survival. For these reasons, Medicare and Medicaid did not cover transplants for chronic hepatitis B.

Current medical treatments (HBIG and lamivudine) have dramatically improved results, and patients with hepatitis B now enjoy the same outcome as patients transplanted for other liver diseases. This turnaround has been so dramatic that in December 1999 Medicare approved chronic hepatitis B as an indication for transplant.

Pre-transplant patients go through a difficult time. They suffer from a variety of symptoms, including jaundice, sleeplessness, itching, fluid buildup, mental confusion, and hemorrhaging. A successful transplant cures these symptoms, and the patient goes on to lead a full, productive life.

This chapter covers the following topics:

- Liver Transplantation: A Brief History
- When Do You Need a Liver Transplant?
    A Common Diagnosis: Hepatitis B
    Signs That You Need a Transplant
    Denial of Transplants
    Paying for Transplants
- The Transplant Team
- Waiting for a Liver
    The Evaluation Process
    The Waiting List
    Transplant Support Groups
- Liver Transplant Surgery
    Donor Livers
    Living-Donor Liver Transplant
    The Surgical Procedure
    The Hospital Stay
- Living with a New Liver
    Medications to Prevent Rejection
    Managing Complications
    Psychological Transformation
- Improved Survival Rates
- How Organs Are Allocated
    UNOS
    Centers of Excellence

Liver Transplantation: A Brief History

The first liver transplant was performed by Dr. Thomas Starzl in 1963 at the University of Colorado in Denver. In 1983, a National Institutes of Health (NIH) consensus conference on the therapeutic role of liver transplantation concluded, "After extensive review and consideration . . . liver transplantation is a therapeutic modality for end-stage liver disease that deserves broader application."

At that time, only six centers in North America and four in Europe performed liver transplantation. Ten years later, 3,442 patients had the procedure at 88 centers in the United States. As of December 1, 2000, there were over 16,000 patients on the active U.S. waiting list.

When Do You Need a Liver Transplant?

A Common Diagnosis: Hepatitis B. Liver transplantation is the most successful therapy for patients with a wide array of diseases that ultimately result in liver failure. Based on 1999 UNOS Organ Procurement Transplant Network data, 9.1 percent of people who had liver transplants were positive for hepatitis B surface antigen. Even more striking, 23 percent of all the recipients were positive for hepatitis B core antibody. Thus, nearly one-quarter of all liver recipients had prior exposure to the hepatitis B virus.

Signs That You Need a Transplant. Obvious clinical signs and symptoms usually accompany advanced liver disease, including:

- ascites (accumulation of fluid in the abdomen)
- encephalopathy (alteration of mental function)
- variceal hemorrhage (bleeding from veins in the esophagus or stomach)
- worsening nutritional status
- diminishing quality of life

> I was having lots of bleeds. One time, I had a bleed during a CT scan. I had to swallow this stuff, and when I threw it up, my veins burst. They did a code blue on me.
>
> My wife told me I was bleeding like a faucet. They tried to keep her in the emergency waiting room, but she said, "If my husband is going to die, I want to be with him."

*I only had to wait nine months for my liver. I have a guardian angel,
my mom who died twelve years ago. She's watching out for me.*

Rick

Patients who have a spontaneous infection in the ascites fluid, low serum albumin (< 2.8 grams/deciliter), clotting problems (prothrombin time > 5 seconds prolonged), and severe sustained jaundice should be given urgent consideration for transplantation. All of the above findings indicate severe liver dysfunction and are late signs of end-stage liver disease.

Many people with cirrhosis have few or no findings of liver disease. Doctors say that these patients have "compensated" cirrhosis, and that it may be too early to consider liver transplantation. However, the waiting list for liver transplants is expanding, while the pool of donors is staying about the same. Patients often wait on the list for one, two, or more years before they get a liver.

Once you have cirrhosis, your doctor must monitor your blood tests closely and watch for any physical signs of "decompensation" in order to time the referral for liver transplantation. Unfortunately, not all patients with compensated cirrhosis are the same; some will remain stable for several years, but others may deteriorate relatively rapidly.

The course of hepatitis B varies greatly, so your physician must make an imperfect estimate of your chances of having a life-threatening complication over a one- to two-year follow-up period. If your doctor estimates that you have more than a 10 percent chance of sustaining such a complication, you should be evaluated for transplantation.

Denial of Transplants. You will be denied a liver transplant if you have AIDS, incurable cancer, active infection in the blood, active alcohol abuse, or severe underlying heart, lung, or multi-organ disease. If you have had prior extensive abdominal surgery, a clotted portal vein, extensive liver cancer, an isolated liver cancer larger than five centimeters, or cancer of the bile ducts, you might be excluded from transplantation.

Paying for Transplants. See Chapter 7, Taking Care of Yourself Financially.

The Transplant Team

Liver transplantation is a complex procedure requiring many specialists to care for you. Usually, your transplant team consists of a hepatologist, a hepatology nurse, a transplant surgeon, a transplant anesthesiologist, a transplant nurse coordinator (who keeps you informed and tells you when a liver becomes available), a social worker (who provides you and your family with emotional support), a psychiatrist (who meets with you and your family to evaluate your strengths and weaknesses and make recommendations to help you through the transplant experience), a nutritionist (who deals with pre-transplant issues, such as overweight problems or nutritional wasting, and helps with recommendations for your post-transplant nutritional needs), and a financial coordinator.

Waiting for a Liver

The Evaluation Process. You will be asked to take many diagnostic tests and meet with a psychiatrist and social worker. Usually, you meet with each person on the transplant team. The process can take a couple of days. When all the tests and interviews are completed, the team meets to approve or deny your candidacy for transplantation and may suggest additional evaluations or consultations.

In trying to evaluate your ability to tolerate transplant surgery, the transplant team will give you some diagnostic tests. Depending on your condition, the tests may include blood tests, colonoscopy (view of the entire colon through a colonoscope), CT scan (a radiologic test that lets doctors see the anatomy and size of your liver), ECG (an electrocardiogram), endoscopy (a procedure that allows doctors to look for ulcers or bleeding in the esophagus or stomach), ERCP (a procedure performed when there is concern about blockage or narrowing in the bile ducts), flexible sigmoidoscopy (a procedure that lets the physician look at the lower colon for polyps, hemorrhoids, ulcers, and colon or rectal cancer), pulmonary function tests (a breathing test that measures the function of your lungs), and ultrasound (a test that gives information about the size and shape of your liver through sound waves). If you have conditions that require additional tests, you may be asked to meet with a consultant, such as a cardiologist.

The Waiting List. Once you're placed on the list, you can wait from a few months to more than two years for a donor liver. This is an incredibly difficult period of waiting apprehensively while having to deal with life changes, physical symptoms, and financial changes. If you're the major breadwinner who can't go to work, you may lose the social network from your job.

It's Catch-22. My enzyme levels have remained rock solid for three years. I can't work. I'm on disability, but unless I can get a hepatitis B liver, they won't move me on the priority list. I have to get sicker in order to get "weller."

Some people, when they get diagnosed with cirrhosis, drop into a decline. Within a year, they're in the hospital. Others stay reasonably healthy, level out, decline slightly, then level out, over and over again. That's me.

Almost my entire family has died in the years I've been sick and placed on the transplant list. I only have one brother left. I've been to eight family funerals—my mother, father, aunts, uncles. They all thought they'd bury ME.

My brother says he can't believe I'm still around. And he teases me all the time. "Nothing will kill you," he says, kidding. "I'll never collect on those insurance policies!"

I struggle with the diagnosis of cirrhosis. It's a spiritual struggle. Every day I have to go to bed and hope someone dies so I can live.

But I've finally gone beyond that. You just have to let go. When it's time—it's time.

One of the most frustrating things is that people who love and care about me ask me if I've heard anything about getting a liver. When you hear that fifty times a day, it gets frustrating. I feel like yelling, "When they cut me, you'll hear about it!"

My family name is Drowning Bear. It goes a long way back to when our tribe was taken to Oklahoma on the Trail of Tears. I dream of bears many times every month.

While I was waiting for a liver, my wife and I took a ride and saw a bear. He took his time and crossed the road right in front of our car. It happened again two weeks later.

Then a bear came to our house. He was hurt. Obviously, he had been in a fight because he had an eye wound that was healing. That bear came right up on our sundeck and ripped open a bag of sunflower seeds we had been saving for the birds. And that started the bears coming to our house—big bears, small bears.

It made us feel really good. Bears are highly respected and revered by almost all tribes. We believe they carry healing power. We felt that those medicine bears were coming to tell us that everything would be all right.

It's critical at this stage to talk about your struggles with a good friend or therapist. Keeping a personal journal is helpful. You are going through a fundamental shift in how you think of yourself and preparing for the psychological changes of the transplant.

Transplant Support Groups. Transplant support groups can be a source of strength and encouragement for pre- and post-transplant patients. The long waiting period, difficult symptoms, the trauma of surgery, the psychological shift of accepting another person's organ—all of these issues are unique to transplant patients. No one else can truly understand what it's like.

I feel a lot more comfortable in the support group now than I did six months ago. Getting to know the people, being involved with their lives, and caring for each other helped.

When people get their transplants, it's like day and night. I look at myself as night, and they're day. Sam, he just got his. I watched him go through his struggle, and he looked really bad. It's amazing what a new liver can do for a person. It's a shot in the arm. Their facial expressions change. They glow.

It helped me to see others waiting. I was a basket case, but I began to accept that it was going to happen. I'd get my liver.

I cried at the group the first time I went. To see all those people—it was overwhelming. For the first time, my husband felt positive about the transplant. He had been reluctant to have me go through it, but he saw so many people looking so good and doing so well.

I think everyone should be required to go to a transplant support group. At first, I dug my heels in and refused to go. I had the feeling I was assisting Mother Nature and wondered whether I had the right to do that. When I saw others in the support group, I decided if I could have that quality of life back, I'd go for it.

Your transplant team can refer you to a support group, or you can check the resources listed at the end of this chapter (also see Resource section at the end of this book). In addition to support groups, many people tell me they find it helpful to read about other liver transplant patients' experiences and about the procedure itself. Here are some books about transplantation and organ donation that my patients recommend:

Resources:

Green, Reg. *The Nicholas Effect, A Boy's Gift to the World*. Sepastopol: O'Reilly, 1999.

Maier, Frank with Ginny Maier. *Sweet Reprieve*. New York: Crown, 1991.

McCartney, Scott. *Defying the Gods*. New York: Macmillan, 1994.

Schomaker, Mary Zimmeth. *Life Line, How One Night Changed Five Lives*. Far Hills: New Horizon, 1996.

Starzl, Thomas E. *The Puzzle People*. Pittsburgh: University of Pittsburgh, 1992.

Liver Transplant Surgery

Donor Livers. Liver transplantation is made possible only through the act of organ donation. In most states, you can sign an organ donor permission statement on your driver's license; a witnessed signature is a legal form of consent. Most organ procurement organizations, however, request additional consent from the closest living relative. These organizations identify potential donors by interacting with emergency rooms and intensive care units.

Organ donation is one of the highest forms of giving and caring, and the vast majority of religious denominations endorse it. The generosity of organ donation makes possible the miracle of transplantation. Here is Judy Ferrin's story:

> At the hospital, the doctors diagnosed my daughter, Allison, with toxic shock syndrome. She went from laughing and joking with me to sleeping, a coma, and dying within 24 hours. She was 19 years old.
>
> Just three weeks before, the two of us were watching a little boy on TV who needed a new heart. We decided to donate our organs if something happened to us—so I knew what her wishes were, and I told her nurse.
>
> The night before the funeral, I tossed and turned. I felt a need to speak at the service, but I was so afraid. We got a call from the doctor

that morning. They had successfully transplanted her kidneys. Other organs were also transplanted, but that was the first, the turning point. A wave of relief went over me. And I was able to speak about Allison to the hundreds of people who came to mourn with our family.

When we give to other people, it helps us through our grief. It helps us as much as the people we give to.

Did you know that the liver donor usually donates as many as seven vascular organs for seven different patients? Suitable liver donors are patients under age 65 who are brain-dead but whose hearts are beating. (In some cases, donors as old as 80 have been used.) They have no underlying malignancy, and they test negative for AIDS and active hepatitis B. The donors must have stable heart function with acceptable liver tests, serum sodium less than 170, and preferably been hospitalized for fewer than seven days. Donors and recipients must match by blood type and approximate body size but not by gender. It's customary to biopsy the donor liver to be certain that it is not scarred, fatty, or severely damaged. Once recovered, the donated organs are flushed with a special solution that preserves them for up to 48 hours.

Patients frequently ask whether organs from donors who test positive for hepatitis B can be used for transplantation. Organs from donors who test positive for surface antigen are usually rejected. Organs from donors who test negative for surface antigen but positive for core antibody or surface antibody may be used. However, the risk of a recipient developing active hepatitis B from a donor positive for core antibody is approximately 50 percent. In the latter circumstance, transplant centers typically treat recipients with either HBIG, lamivudine, or both, to prevent recurrence of hepatitis B post-transplant. Because of this risk, livers from core antibody-positive donors are typically restricted to recipients who already have hepatitis B infection or who are critically ill. The latter patients need urgent transplantation and are listed at high UNOS (United Network for Organ Sharing) status. (For more information on UNOS, see Resources at the end of this chapter.)

Despite efforts to use all potential donor organs, we currently face a crisis in supply and availability of donor organs. We encourage all readers of this book to work with their local organ procurement organizations to increase the public awareness of the critical need and value of organ donation. It's important for all family members to discuss organ and tissue donation. Everyone should consider signing a Uniform Donor Card.

Resource: For more information on organ donation, contact the Coalition on Donation, an alliance of national organizations and local coalitions that educates the public about organ donation at 804-330-8620. Email: coalition@unos.org Website: www.shareyourlife.org

How can we as physicians attempt to deal with the crisis in availability of donor organs? The cadaveric supply of donor livers has remained relatively constant at about 4000 to 4500 donor livers each year for the last five years. The current U.S. waiting list is over 16,000.

We need to increase the donor pool in innovative ways in order to meet the expanding need for donor organs. Use of older donors, livers with increased amounts of fat, hepatitis C antibody-positive livers, and hepatitis B core antibody-positive livers has failed to substantially expand the donor pool. Splitting of cadaveric livers for use in two recipients works well for a pediatric (left lateral segment) and adult recipient (right lobe + left medial segment); splits for two adult recipients works less well. For this reason, our center and many others have embarked upon the use of adult living donors (right lobe donation) for adults.

Living-Donor Liver Transplant. You may be thinking, "By the time I need a transplant, there will be too many people on the waiting list, and I won't ever get one!" One solution for the shortage of donors may be living-donor liver transplantation, where a portion of a living donor's liver is removed and then transplanted. The Japanese, for example, still debate the concept of brain death, so most liver donations in Japan are from live donors. In the past, the majority of live donor transplant operations were performed in pediatric recipients. In the U.S., however, more live donor liver transplants now are performed in adults.

At the time of this writing, the University of Colorado has performed 50 adult-to-adult live-donor liver transplants. The vast majority have been between relatives, although close friends and personal relationships may be considered. All donors are alive and tolerated the liver resection. Their livers regenerated back to normal size within 16 weeks.

We recently evaluated the impact of partial liver donation on the quality of life of the living donors:

- 75 % of donors had complete recovery and returned to normal life within an average of 3.4 months after surgery.
- 96 % returned to work at an average of 2.4 months.

- 42 % described a change in body image related to the scar from the incision.
- 71 % had mild ongoing abdominal discomfort.

Personal relationships between donor and recipient were the same or better in 96 percent of cases. The relationship of the donor to his or her life partner was the same or better in 80 percent of cases. Most donors reported out-of-pocket expenses not covered by insurance plans. All patients reported that under the same circumstances they would donate again, and 96 percent of the donors felt that they benefited from the experience.

Survival and rates of retransplantation in recipients of living-donor liver transplants are similar to results after cadavaric transplants. Biliary complications occur more frequently compared to standard cadaveric transplantation. However, because of the critical lack of cadaveric donor livers, it is my opinion that living-donor donation for adults will become increasingly common in the United States.

In our program, we have developed selection criteria for both donor and recipient. Our current criteria for selection of recipients center around two concepts. First, we feel that recipients should have an excellent chance for favorable post-transplant outcome. Second, the recipient should be in urgent need of a transplant for survival and might die while waiting for standard cadaveric transplantation

Donors for living donor liver transplantation must be relatively young (less than 50 years old), normal body size, healthy without medical problems, and they cannot have a history of prior abdominal surgery. Donors and recipients should have compatible blood types and an emotional bond. Unlike other transplants, livers do not need to be matched by tissue type. The donor liver, however, must be of sufficient size that the right lobe will be large enough for the recipient.

The living donor undergoes careful medical, psychological, and social evaluation. Potential donors may be rejected because their livers are unsuitable or they have underlying medical conditions that increase the risk of complications from surgery.

By the time Jim was diagnosed, his hepatitis B was very advanced. The doctors told him he had months, not years, before he would need a transplant. "You won't make the wait," they said. "You'd better get a living donor."

Several members of our family volunteered to be living donors, but two nephews failed because their livers were deformed. Jim's brother-in-law had heart trouble. Even a good friend offered, but she was a tiny woman, and you have to be bigger than the patient.

Then Jim was hospitalized; he was so sick. The doctors came in at midnight and said that they had a cadaver liver for him. I feel so lucky that we were pulled back from the brink!

Deanne

Risk to the donor is small, but present. The current estimate of the risk of death is 1 in 500 liver donations. Other complications can occur, however, including pulmonary emboli, gastrointestinal bleeding, bile duct injury, and infection. The overall complication rate in donors is 10 percent, with postoperative biliary leak the most common problem. The liver is the only internal human organ that regenerates and renews itself; the portion of the liver that is removed regenerates over 8 to 16 weeks.

The overall outcome for recipients primarily relates to their pre-transplant clinical condition. When the procedure is performed in stable patients under non-urgent conditions, the one-year survival rate is greater than 90 percent. Survival rates decrease when the transplant takes place in more urgent circumstances. It is likely that living-donor liver transplantation will become commonplace in the future, and selection criteria will change.

The Surgical Procedure. The human body has two kidneys, two lungs—but only one liver. Scientists have created artificial kidneys (kidney dialysis) and even artificial hearts, but no one has been able to duplicate the hundreds of functions of the liver to create an effective liver dialysis machine. Liver transplant surgery, therefore, has no fallback position, no margin for error.

The call for my transplant came in the middle of the night. I was told I had a couple of hours to get to the hospital. I live in the mountains, and we were just ahead of a huge snowstorm coming in. There was no traffic. The flakes were just starting. We breezed right into the city.

All during that fall, I appreciated the blue sky, the Aspens. I spent a lot of quiet time by myself, and I felt that I had the courage to give the transplant a try. I used that time to learn to have confidence in the doctors and the hospital.

It was all right for me to die. I had to be a realist. My veins constantly had to be injected to avoid bleeds, and I was wasting away—so thin I could hardly turn over in bed. I was at peace.

When we arrived at the hospital, I didn't hesitate. I wasn't afraid—I really wasn't. The surgery began at 7 a.m. and finished by noon.

Helena

Although the original method pioneered by Dr. Starzl has been modified, the basic technique remains essentially unchanged. The operation has three phases:

1. dissection to access the patient's liver
2. removal of the patient's liver
3. connecting the donated liver

First, the surgeon meticulously dissects tissues and promptly controls bleeding vessels to expose the patient's liver. This process takes about one to two hours. Blood loss ranges from zero to five pints of red blood cells.

In the next phase, the surgeon clamps the blood vessels supplying your liver and removes the liver. Then the surgeon and anesthesiologist work together to maintain adequate blood clotting factors. The anesthesiologist carefully monitors your blood and blood pressure to give you the proper fluids and blood products. In the last phase, the surgeon positions the donor liver in your abdomen and sews the blood vessels together. This procedure takes from one-and-a-half to three hours; blood loss ranges from zero to five pints.

Once all the vessels are connected, the surgeon must unclamp the main vessels. After unclamping, one of the more critical periods of the procedure begins—especially if your blood clotting is poor. After you stabilize, your surgeon connects your bile duct to the donor bile duct and removes the donor gallbladder.

Livers typically begin to function immediately after their blood supply is established. Clotting improves, and the liver makes bile on the operating table!

"The most critical moment in the operation," says University of Colorado's Chief of Transplantation, Dr. Igal Kam, "is when we release the clamps holding the vessels going to the new liver, and the new liver changes in color from pale or dark brown to a more pink-brown, because new blood is flowing to the liver. When we see the yellow-brown bile start to appear from the bile duct, we can relax because we know the liver is going to work. There's no room for mistakes in this procedure.

"About 40 to 50 percent of patients go off the respirator in the operating room and we can talk to them. After six to eight hours of surgery, it's great to talk to the patient. We deal with very sick people who sometimes have only hours to live. After the transplant, then we see the miracle."

The Hospital Stay. After the operation you may be monitored in an intensive care unit (ICU) where the staff is specifically trained to manage this early post-transplant period. Patients who are very stable may bypass the ICU and transfer from recovery room directly to the transplant inpatient floor. If you are transferred to ICU and have no complications, you'll spend 24 to 48 hours in the ICU and then transfer to the inpatient transplant unit.

Usually, patients stay in the hospital from five to 20 days depending on their condition. Some patients require extensive rehabilitation, such as physical therapy or nursing, due to their weakened situation before the transplant.

After discharge you'll be monitored in transplant outpatient clinics for a few weeks to a few months and then you'll return to the care of your referring primary care physician or gastroenterologist. The transplant center continues to guide patient management through close cooperation with referring physicians.

Living with a New Liver

Although highly variable from patient to patient, most people require from three to six months to physically recover from surgery and adjust to new medications. An inspiration to transplant athletes, Chris Klug, a 28-year-old American snowboarder, took the gold in the World Cup parallel giant slalom on January 17, 2001—less than nine months after his liver transplant for primary sclerosing cholangitis!

Liver transplantation is a profound event that affects every part of a patient's life—the mind as well as the body. Patients must learn to live with lifelong medications, deal with the fear of rejection of the organ, and come to terms with a profound physical and psychological transformation.

Transplant is an intense experience—physically, mentally, spiritually. When I got that call for my liver, all those feelings of guilt, anger, and fear started racing through me. After the transplant, I heard the doctors talking. They were about to give me supermeds to fight off rejection.

I started praying for acceptance. Then I started talking to my new liver and welcoming it. I said, "Welcome aboard. I love you. I'm really scared, but you're a part of me now. You're a part of the engine, and you're not just along for the ride."

It worked. I never needed the supermeds.

Carl

Medications to Prevent Rejection. After the transplant, you need to take medications for the rest of your life to prevent your immune system from rejecting your new liver. The medications are called immunosuppressants and include the following: cyclosporine (Sandimmune®, Neoral®), tacrolimus (Prograf®), sirolimus (Rapamune®), azathioprine (Imuran®), steroids (Prednisone®, Solumedrol®), and mycophenolate mofetil (Cellcept®).

Most patients take either cyclosporine, tacrolimus, or sirolimus as primary therapy, and use the other agents to strengthen the anti-rejection effect. In the first six to 12 months it's common to take two or three anti-rejection medications. After that period most patients remain on cyclosporine, tacrolimus, or sirolimus, either alone or in combination with low-dose Prednisone®.

Although the medications have side effects, most of them are dose-related and respond to either lowering the dose of the specific immunosuppressant or changing to another medication.

Never change doses by yourself. All dose adjustments of immunosuppressants require the supervision of your doctor. If you take too little immunosuppression, you run the risk of rejecting your liver transplant. If you take too much immunosuppression, you risk adverse reactions to medications [infection, renal failure, hypertension, hyperlipidemia (excess blood cholesterol and fat), diabetes mellitus].

Managing Complications. It's essential that your transplant team supervise you closely during your post-transplant outpatient care. The most concerning problems that can occur in patients with hepatitis B are rejection and recurrence of hepatitis B.

If rejection occurs, it typically does so within the first three months of the transplant and is detected by a rise in liver enzymes. Elevations of liver enzymes and bilirubin occur, although the first change noted is usually an increase in AST. In some cases, rejection is very mild and does not require additional immunosuppressive treatment. In more severe cases of rejection, the patient may experience fever (up to 102°F), poor appetite, fatigue, and malaise.

Nearly all rejections occur within three months of transplantation, but occasionally rejection happens later. "Late rejection" usually results from low levels of immunosuppressive therapy due to improper dosing, addition of a new medication, or development of a simultaneous illness such as diarrhea or liver dysfunction. Rejection usually responds to intravenous steroids or other strategies (OKT3).

Recurrent episodes of hepatitis B are relatively rare due to current post-transplant treatment with HBIG and lamivudine. Nonetheless, hepatitis B can recur and may be mistaken for rejection. Accurate diagnosis is essential because aggressive anti-rejection treatments, such as high-dose steroids and OKT3, may worsen hepatitis B and predispose the patient to fibrosing cholestatic hepatitis (a rapidly progressive form of hepatitis B that can lead to graft loss and patient death). Recurrent hepatitis B must be carefully considered before one embarks on a course to treat rejection.

> *Ray was just fine until four months after his transplant. He started feeling bad again, and his labs went way up. We were worried that it was the hepatitis B coming back, even though Ray takes lamivudine and HBIG shots. But the doctors thought it was rejection. They gave him intravenous Prednisone—a huge dose for three days in a row.*
>
> *Yesterday, the labs went down, so I guess they caught it in time. They told us that rejection can happen any time—even 20 or 30 years from now. It's very common, and they don't get so concerned. The doctors are calm; they deal with it. If the Prednisone blast doesn't work, they have other meds.*
>
> *Patti*

HBIG is given in high doses initially and typically once a month for life, thereafter. This treatment inactivates hepatitis B and leads to long-term remission. Recently, lamivudine has been used with increasing frequency by transplant centers and its use may decrease or eliminate the need for HBIG.

When hepatitis B recurs, patients usually don't have symptoms and doctors detect it as an increase in blood levels of liver enzymes as early as one week after the transplant. Recurrent hepatitis B is often confused with rejection since the histologic features of rejection and hepatitis B on liver biopsies overlap considerably. However, positive surface antigen or HBV DNA is presumptive evidence for active hepatitis B. Transplant centers treat patients based upon these test results, clinical impression, and experience.

Recurrent hepatitis B can be a serious problem, resulting in severe liver injury and loss of the transplanted graft. Fortunately, this is now an extremely rare event due to effective therapeutic strategies to prevent hepatitis B infection of the graft.

Psychological Transformation. Post-transplant patients go through a period of accepting the "gift of life." The feelings are common to everyone and include curiosity about the donor, feelings of guilt that someone had to die so they could live, and a sense of indebtedness—of feeling overwhelmed and struggling with how to repay an enormous gift.

Michael Talamantes, transplant social worker at the University of Colorado Health Sciences Center, says that patients often write a letter of thanks to the donor's family. The donor's identity is kept confidential, so the letter is sent through official channels. If the donor's family members wish to reply, they will. And if not, it's important to respect their privacy.

Four people were transplanted the same night: two kidneys, lungs, and a liver—all from the same donor, a 17-year-old boy.

It took my wife and me a couple of months to compose a letter that said the right things. We tried to make the donor's family feel that they had made the right decision. We told them they gave me the gift of life, and that their son continued to live in all the people who received organ donations from him.

We didn't hear for months. They finally wrote. It was the most beautiful letter—and it put our hearts at peace.

Lee

Feelings of guilt over the donor's death take time to work through. Although it seems obvious that the donor's death is independent of your need for a liver, the feelings are almost universal.

The sense of indebtedness is often overwhelming. Some people do community service or visit patients in the hospital who are awaiting transplants. Every patient is touched in some way.

> *I feel so much gratitude for all the doctors. Now I understand how hard they have to work to get you your liver and to do the transplant.*
>
> *I sat down for two days and wrote thank-you letters to every doctor Ralph had. I want them to know how grateful I am for saving my husband's life.*
>
> Nan

As in every new experience, you may have contradictory feelings. It's important to pay attention to them. Whatever normal, contradictory feelings you have, you need to sort through them to adjust to your new sense of yourself. To complicate matters, you may get mixed messages from others. Are you a hero, a biotechnological miracle, or does your boss see you as damaged goods, a drain on the company's health insurance? Whatever your experiences, they are profound indeed. You are not alone in wrestling with these issues.

> *I have two grandchildren born since my transplant—and I'm alive to enjoy them.*

> *When I returned to work after my transplant, people were apprehensive and leery of me. They expected me to be down-and-out. I'd hear whispers, "Shouldn't he be home? His hands are shaking." And I'd think, if you were on all these medicines, your hands would be shaking, too.*

> *I consider myself very fortunate to still be here and enjoy my family. After an experience like a transplant, you need to concentrate on what's important to you—family, family, family.*

> *Why am I so happy? The bleeds I had before my transplant made me appreciate every day. Now I've got a second life!*

My quality of life post-transplant is just amazing. I probably don't have more money. In fact, I'm making less money, but my relationships are better.

I've got my son back. He was 15 at the time, and he was so afraid he would lose me that he pulled back emotionally. Now he's 21, and we're moving to a new level as father and son, a more adult relationship.

Having a terminal illness makes you look at your life. Am I here just so I can be sick or die? Or is there something beyond that?

After I get a transplant, I'll take some time to repair and adjust. I want to work with people who have HIV or children who are starving. After I went to Vietnam, and even as a kid, I had this dream about going into the Peace Corps. There's something inside me that says I can help somehow.

The wonderful thing about transplants is that we're all connected. My liver may have come from someone with a different lifestyle, race, or religion. Like Martin Luther King said, "We live together as brothers or perish together as fools."

Improved Survival Rates

The heartening news for patients with chronic hepatitis B is that survival rates have dramatically improved due to advances in antiviral therapy, immunosuppression (beginning with cyclosporine in 1979), and the team approach to liver transplantation. Before cyclosporine, patients were treated with high doses of Prednisone and azathioprine. Procedures, such as thoracic duct drainage, splenectomy, and anti-lymphocyte immunoglobulin injections, were used to further suppress the immune system and prevent rejection. Before 1979, results were poor: 32 percent of patients survived one year and only 22 percent survived 30 months.

The picture has changed dramatically. Liver transplant results show that average one- and three-year patient survival rates in the U.S. from 1988 to 1995 were 77 and 68 percent respectively. During the same period the average one- and three-year survival rates in Europe were 73 and 65 percent. Our results at the University of Colorado compared favorably to the overall results in both the U.S. and Europe: one- and three-year patient survival rates were 86 and 78 percent. Currently, survival of hepatitis B patients is similar to non-hepatitis B patients undergoing liver transplantation (see Figure 9A).

The reality is, however, that not all patients survive. Deaths occurring within the first six months are due to nonfunction of the donor's liver, clotting of the main artery to the liver, infection, multi-organ failure, or rejection. When deaths occur later after the transplant, they are more commonly due to malignancy or complications of atherosclerosis (hardening of the arteries) and rarely to rejection or infection.

The outlook is very hopeful. We anticipate that current immunosuppressive protocols will reduce adverse metabolic effects and continue to improve the long-term outlook for transplant recipients. (Since 1995 one-year survival rates at the University of Colorado exceed 90 percent.) Our ultimate goal, of course, is to restore you to your normal life.

How Organs Are Allocated

UNOS. In the United States, the United Network for Organ-Sharing (UNOS) regulates the distribution or allocation of donor organs. Here's how it works.

The United States is divided into 11 regions for organ procurement and allocation. Several local organ procurement organizations (OPOs) exist within each region. When a patient is approved for transplantation, he or she is placed on local, regional, and national waiting lists. Typically, more than 80 percent of recipients receive organs from local donors.

As waiting lists continue to expand, will a shortage of donors lead to increasing numbers of people dying while they wait for a liver? Although the number of patients listed more than quintupled from 1988 to 1998—and the number of liver transplants only doubled—the waiting list mortality rate of approximately 8 percent did not change. Two factors kept the waiting list mortality relatively constant during this period: earlier listing and transplantation at more urgent UNOS status. Mortality rate on the waiting list is now beginning to rise.

Centers of Excellence. UNOS displays the results for liver transplantation in the United States on its continually updated Website (www.unos.org). Patient and graft survivals for one- and three-year outcomes are given in combined totals and for each individual center. Results are also adjusted for differences in patient populations according to variables known to influence outcome after liver transplantation: UNOS listing status, diagnosis of fulminant hepatic failure, age, renal

FIGURE 9A: PATIENT SURVIVAL AFTER LIVER TRANSPLANTATION FOR CHRONIC HEPATITIS B.

% OF PATIENTS SURVIVING

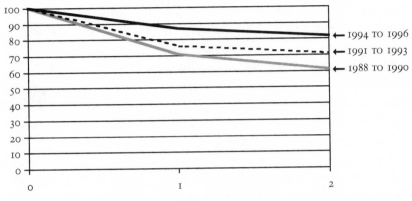

YEARS AFTER TRANSPLANT

LEGEND 9A: The survival of patients transplanted for chronic hepatitis B has improved dramatically over the last decade, primarily due to widespread use of HBIG. Patients transplanted in the time interval between 1988 and 1990 had a two-year survival of 61%, but those transplanted more recently, between 1994 to 1996, had a two-year survival of 82%. The survival rates for chronic hepatitis B patients transplanted between 1994 and 1996 were comparable or better than survival of those transplanted for non-hepatitis B indications. Outcomes have continued to improve since 1996. The data for this figure were taken from a publication of the American Liver Foundation: Vierling, J.M., L.W. Teperman, A.P. Brownstein. *Hepatitis B: An Appropriate Indication for Liver Transplantation.* December 1998. (See also Vierling, J.M., L.W. Teperman, A.P. Brownstein. *Hepatitis B and Liver Transplantation.* Seminars in Liver Disease 2000;20:1S-35S).

failure, presence of hepatitis B, and presence of primary liver cancer. Using this stratification method, results from each center can be compared to the expected outcome.

Intuitively, one could suggest that this analysis identifies true "centers of excellence," because it is based solely upon adjusted medical outcomes. Unfortunately, this criteria has not surfaced as the most relevant factor when negotiating contracts with third-party insurers.

Medicare was the first to put into practice the concept of centers of excellence in liver transplantation. Additional third-party insurers, such as Blue Cross/Blue Shield, Prudential, United Resource Network, and Kaiser Permanente use similar criteria. With the explosion of HMOs, the criteria for designating centers of excellence are more of a mixture of medical outcome and economic impact. Adoption of standardized medical criteria for designation of "centers of excellence" would eliminate the potential that a given program could be an insurer's transplant center by simply offering the lowest price.

Many people have suggested that the current number of 117 transplant programs is far in excess of what the donor organ pool can provide. More than half the programs in the U.S. perform fewer than 20 liver transplants per year; 75 percent of all liver transplants are performed by only 25 percent of the programs.

A recent publication by UNOS in *The New England Journal of Medicine* confirms that transplant teams that perform more than 20 transplants per year achieve optimal patient and graft survival. According to this analysis, the chance to die after liver transplantation is almost twice as great when the transplant is done by a program performing fewer than 20 transplants per year. Because more than half the programs in the U.S. perform fewer than 20 transplants a year, one must question the wisdom of encouraging proliferation of transplant centers.

Some states have invoked the concept of "certification of need" to ensure a balance between the regional need for transplantation and the number of transplant centers. Further increases in the number of transplant centers should be discouraged unless dictated by regional requirements.

Resource: Call the toll-free UNOS patient information number at 1-888-TXINFO1 (1-888-894-6361). Website: www.unos.org To request free single copies of the following brochures, call or write to UNOS, P.O. Box 13770, Richmond, VA 23286-2659: *What Every Patient Needs to Know; Information for Patients; Share Your Life. Share Your Decision*SM*; Vital Connections.*

Resource: Updated Waitlist and Transplant Summary Reports, statistics by state, region, or individual hospitals, and other information are available on the UNOS Website: www.unos.org. To order free printed versions of the *1997 Report of Center Specific Graft and Patient Survival Rates* by individual volume or complete 7-volume set (there is a shipping charge), contact the UNOS Professional Services Department at 804-330-8541.

Resource: Regional organ recovery organizations are a good source of information. To locate your region's organization, call the UNOS patient information number listed above.

Resource: For information on national organizations and local coalitions that educate the public about organ donation, call the Coalition on Donation, 804-330-8620. Email: coalition@unos.org Website: www.shareyourlife.org You may also request a free brochure on organ donation from the Coalition on Donation by calling 1-800-355-SHARE.

Resource: For a free Transplant Support Group Directory (of more than 300 pre- and post-transplant support groups nationwide) and a sample copy of the *Solstice* newsletter (dedicated to organ transplantation), call Chronimed Pharmacy: 1-800-888-5753 and ask for a patient specialist.

Resource: For free pamphlets and information about transplants and organ donation, call a nationwide support group for transplant patients and their families, Transplant Recipients International Organization (TRIO): 1-800-TRIO-386.

Resource: A uniform donor card is enclosed in this book. Discuss organ and tissue donation with family members. After completing and signing the Uniform Donor Card, be sure to have your signature witnessed by two people.

To every thing there is a season, and a time to every purpose under the heaven...

A time to weep, and a time to laugh; a time to mourn, and a time to dance...

Ecclesiastes

1 0

LIVER CANCER
Are You At Risk?

I was diagnosed in the early '80s with a death sentence—10 to 15 years to live. I was 24.

At the time, there was no interferon or lamivudine. I didn't have any complications for ten years until my enzymes skyrocketed. Interferon was available by then. I went e-antigen negative but still showed virus on a PCR, so I'm on EPIVIR® now.

My liver seems to be okay, but I'm still at risk for cancer. And my insurance will only pay for a cancer check once a year. Well, I knew I could die, but at least I've lived to age 42!

Carter

THE INCIDENCE OF LIVER cancer, also known as hepatocellular carcinoma (HCC) or hepatoma, is increasing both worldwide and in the United States. The major risk factor for liver cancer is cirrhosis due to chronic viral hepatitis from both hepatitis B virus (HBV) and hepatitis C virus (HCV).

The risk factor was discovered in the 1970s by R. Palmer Beasley, M.D., who noticed high rates of hepatitis B and liver cancer in Taiwan. Although he faced skepticism, he and his colleagues eventually proved that a virus, hepatitis B, can cause liver cancer.

Worldwide, hepatitis B is the most common cause of liver disease associated with liver cancer. In the United States, the increasing incidence of liver cancer is related mainly to chronic hepatitis C. The reported risk of development of HCC in cirrhotic patients with chronic viral hepatitis ranges from 0.8 to 5.8 percent per year. At an incident rate of 5 percent per year, a patient with cirrhosis would have a cumulative risk of developing liver cancer of 14.3 percent at three years and 22.8 percent at five years.

Patients with chronic hepatitis B who don't have cirrhosis may still be at risk for liver cancer, even though this risk is much lower than that of patients with cirrhosis. The risk is greatest for those patients who acquired hepatitis B via vertical transmission from mother to newborn at the time of delivery. In Taiwan, approximately 50 percent of all liver cancers occur in noncirrhotic patients.

Most of my patients don't realize that hepatitis B can cause liver cancer. But before you panic or worry unnecessarily, consider the following:

1. Only a minority of patients with hepatitis B will ever develop liver cancer.
2. Effective therapies exist for tumors detected early.
3. Liver cancer is almost entirely restricted to those with advanced liver disease who have extensive fibrosis (stage III) or cirrhosis.

Of course, you're wondering if you are in danger. This chapter provides you with information regarding risk factors, warning signs, screening and diagnostic tests for liver cancer, and results of current treatment. Here are the topics I'll cover:

- Overview: What Is Liver Cancer?
    Primary Liver Cancer
    Secondary Liver Cancer
    Is Primary Liver Cancer on the Rise?
- Common Risk Factors
    Stage of Hepatitis B
    Duration of Infection
    Other Liver Diseases
- Warning Signs
    Asymptomatic but with Underlying Cirrhosis
    Deterioration in Liver Function
    Pain
    Sudden Development of Portal Hypertension
    Other Symptoms

- Testing
  Early Screening Guidelines
      Blood Tests (Serial Measurement of Alpha-fetoprotein)
      Radiologic Imaging
  Diagnostic Tests
- Treatment
  Cancer Staging
      (1) Early Stage
      (2) Advanced Stage
      (3) Metastic Liver Cancer
  Hepatic Resection
  Transplantation
  Chemoembolization
  High-Frequency Radio Waves (Radiofrequency Tumor Ablation)
  Alcohol Injection, Cryosurgery
  Chemotherapy
- Summary

Overview: What Is Liver Cancer?

Primary Liver Cancer (Hepatoma). Primary liver cancer, also known as hepatoma or hepatocellular carcinoma, is a malignant tumor that originates within the liver. Nearly all hepatomas originate from cells composed of the main tissue of the liver (hepatocytes), rather than from cells of the biliary tract, fibrous tissue, blood vessels, or fat.

Secondary Liver Cancer. In the United States, primary liver cancer is relatively rare. Most cancers migrate to the liver, are called secondary cancers, and have their primary site in other organs of the body, such as the colon, breast, or lung. Secondary liver cancers frequently appear as multiple liver masses, while primary liver cancers commonly appear as a solitary mass.

Physicians distinguish secondary from primary liver cancers by imaging the liver (ultrasonography, CT, MRT) and biopsing the tissue. The finding of secondary liver cancer means that tumor cells have traveled far from their primary site, typically indicating a poor chance of survival. Liver transplantation is not indicated for secondary liver cancers.

Is Primary Liver Cancer on the Rise? In the past, primary liver cancers were so rare in the United States that doctors often selected these cases for presentation at medical Grand Rounds lectures. Today, we diagnose primary liver cancer with increasing frequency, especially in patients with chronic hepatitis due to hepatitis B or C. The Centers for Disease Control and Prevention report that the incidence of hepatoma increased from 1.4 to 2.4 per 100,000 people between 1979 and 1995.

In my own state of Colorado, the number of cases of hepatoma doubled from 1986 to 1995. The number of patients with hepatoma presented to the Tumor Board at University Hospital was seven in 1988 and 27 in 1997.

Common Risk Factors

Stage of Hepatitis B. The most important predictor of liver cancer is the condition of the liver tissue (histologic stage). Noncirrhotic patients have low risk, patients with extensive fibrosis (stage III) run an intermediate risk, and those with cirrhosis are at greatest risk. Several studies have examined the risk of developing liver cancer in patients with established cirrhosis due to hepatitis B. The current estimate of the annual incidence of hepatoma is about 2 percent per year. Patients with early cirrhosis probably have a risk of 1 percent per year, and those with advanced established cirrhosis have a risk closer to 5 to 6 percent per year. Patients with hepatitis B and cirrhosis should undergo periodic surveillance with alpha-fetoprotein and ultrasonography every six months.

Noncirrhotic patients without significant fibrosis are at low risk for liver cancer and most do not have to undergo screening for liver tumors. One exception to this guideline is the patient who acquired chronic hepatitis B at the time of birth. Lifetime risk of liver cancer in this group of patients is estimated at 50 percent for men and 20 percent for women. For this reason, screening for liver cancer (see below) is recommended even for noncirrhotic patients who acquired the infection at birth if they have had hepatitis B for 30 years or more.

Patients with cirrhosis run a considerable lifetime risk of developing hepatoma and should undergo screening. Cirrhotic patients who develop sudden onset of decompensation (see Later Warning Signs of Cirrhosis in Chapter 4), should undergo diagnostic studies to rule out liver cancer.

Duration of Infection. Most data suggest that the median time period for developing hepatoma is approximately 30 years from the date of infection or 10 years after the onset of cirrhosis. If you don't have cirrhosis but have had hepatitis B for 30 years, you may still be at risk for liver cancer.

Other Liver Diseases. Any liver disease that hastens the development of cirrhosis may also increase the likelihood of developing hepatoma. The four most common concurrent hepatic diseases in hepatitis B patients that accelerate disease progression are chronic alcohol use, hepatitis C, hepatitis D, and genetic hemochromatosis.

Multiple studies have now conclusively demonstrated that patients with hepatitis B who drink alcohol add fuel to the hepatitis B fire. Chronic daily consumption of alcohol is associated with acceleration to cirrhosis, increased risk for liver failure, increased risk for needing liver transplantation, and increased risk for development of liver cancer. Similar risks have been observed in patients with hepatitis B who are co-infected with hepatitis C. In addition, hemochromatosis, the most common genetic liver disease, causes excessive accumulation of iron in the liver, which also accelerates liver disease due to hepatitis B and therefore potentially increases the risk of liver cancer.

Warning Signs

Asymptomatic but with Underlying Cirrhosis. Many patients develop hepatoma without any changes in symptoms or obvious progression of their disease. That's why I recommend screening tests, such as alpha-fetoprotein and ultrasonography for all patients with bridging fibrosis (stage III) or cirrhosis. Detection of hepatoma with screening tests may result in more effective treatment and better outcomes.

> *I didn't even have time to come to grips with his diagnosis. There was no hope. I got him to the hospital, and they tried to shrink the tumor with chemoembolization, but the tumor had invaded the vena cava. He came home on Wednesday and died on Friday.*
>
> *Trudi*

Deterioration in Liver Function. A stable cirrhotic patient may be fully employed, have normal levels of energy, conduct normal social activities, and have stable liver tests. When such a patient develops hepatoma, liver function may deteriorate for no other apparent reason. Signs of deterioration are increasing fatigue, mental confusion (encephalopathy), fluid retention (ascites, edema), or gastrointestinal bleeding. Alternatively, the patient's liver tests may suddenly deteriorate with rising bilirubin, diminishing clotting factors, increase in liver enzymes, and drop in serum albumin. Some patients experience only a loss of appetite, fever, and unexplained weight loss.

Pain. A tumor can grow rapidly, causing the liver capsule to expand, and tumor cells can invade adjacent nerve roots, blood vessels, and lymphatics. As the hepatoma enlarges and impinges on adjacent structures, it can create significant pain and discomfort. Development of persistent moderate to severe pain in the right upper quadrant of the abdomen in a patient with cirrhosis may point to the diagnosis of hepatoma.

Sudden Development of Portal Hypertension. Hepatoma is a vascular tumor and often invades vascular structures, such as blood or fluid-bearing vessels or ducts. If the tumor enters the portal vein, it may plug the vessel or cause blood clotting that blocks the vein. An acute rise in portal pressure related to this blockage may result in an upper gastrointestinal bleed (variceal hemorrhage), swelling of the abdomen (ascites) or ankles, worsening of existing ascites, development of diuretic-resistant ascites, mental confusion (encephalopathy), or worsening of existing encephalopathy.

Other Symptoms. Patients may attribute certain nonspecific symptoms (fatigue, loss of appetite, poor energy) to their ongoing hepatitis B when the symptoms may be related to the emergence of hepatoma. These patients often delay notifying their physicians for several months. Such a delay may convert a potentially treatable tumor to one that has spread beyond the confines of the liver and may no longer be treatable.

Testing

Early Screening Guidelines. Doctors have not yet established widely-accepted guidelines for screening for hepatoma in patients with hepatitis B. However, recent clinical trials have indicated that screening with both alpha-fetoprotein and ultrasonography detect early tumors and results in improved patient survival. Nonetheless, many of my comments on screening come from my own experience and represent my bias regarding the most cost-effective and sensitive approach to this problem.

The two screening tests doctors use to detect liver cancer are (1) blood tests (serial measurement of alpha-fetoprotein) and (2) radiologic imaging.

1. Blood Tests (Serial Measurement of Alpha-fetoprotein).
Hepatoma cells synthesize a protein called alpha-fetoprotein and release the protein into the bloodstream. A very high alpha-fetoprotein [>500 nanograms (ng) per milliliter (ml)] or a sustained rise in alpha-fetoprotein on serial measurements (with the last value > 150 ng/ml) may predict the development of hepatoma.

However, the accuracy of alpha-fetoprotein alone in predicting hepatoma is poor. Therefore, doctors may order supplemental radiologic tests, biopsies, or even a surgical incision (laparotomy). In addition, 20 to 30 percent of the hepatomas that occur in patients with hepatitis B may lack the ability to produce alpha-fetoprotein. In such cases, the tumors progress undetected by the serial alpha-fetoprotein measurements. Radiologic imaging of the liver is required to screen for these tumors.

2. Radiologic Imaging. Although CT scans and magnetic resonance imaging (MRI) with enhancing agents may be slightly more sensitive than ultrasonography, they are prohibitively expensive for use in screening. Ultrasonography, on the other hand, which can detect the majority of early hepatomas, is much less costly and is the radiologic screening choice. I currently advise both my cirrhotic patients, and noncirrhotic patients who acquired hepatitis at birth and have had disease for 30 years or more, to have alpha-fetoprotein measurements and ultrasonography of the liver every six months.

> *Four years ago, an absolutely routine physical showed there was something wrong with my liver functions. I had chronic active hepatitis B. Within six months I had ascites, terrible swelling. I went on an EPIVIR®/famciclovir study and my viral count went undetectable.*
>
> *About nine months after I started the antivirals, a routine ultrasound showed hepatoma. It was a really big shock!*
>
> *Art*

Diagnostic Tests. If screening tests detect a lesion that might be cancerous, doctors may biopsy the mass with the guidance of ultrasonography or CT. Other imaging studies (CT, MRI, or angiography) can detect early hepatoma in the patient with rising alpha-fetoprotein or worsening of symptoms when ultrasonography fails to reveal a definite lesion. The type of imaging study is ordered at your physician's discretion.

Treatment

Cancer Staging. In order to select proper treatment, the physician must determine the stage of the hepatoma. This is usually done with radiologic imaging, laparoscopy, or abdominal exploratory surgery.

(1) Early Stage. Patients with a solitary tumor less than five centimeters in diameter or patients with up to three tumors, all less than three centimeters in diameter, may be candidates for surgery to remove the tumor (hepatic resection) or liver transplantation. Recurrence of the tumor is common if resection is performed. Cure and excellent long-term survival are the rule with liver transplantation.

> *I was playing around with getting on the liver transplant list, so they gave me an ultrasound. It was okay.*
>
> *Three months later, they did another one and found a hepatoma that had grown to over two centimeters. That's fairly big. But it was located on the surface of the liver. The doctors told me that was a good sign. They decided to try chemoembolization and put me on the transplant list.*
>
> *Harvey*

(2) Advanced Stage. More advanced stages of hepatoma usually represent multiple tumor nodules involving one or both liver lobes. The tumor may have invaded the main liver vessels. Advanced stage tumors have a poorer prognosis, and typically doctors do not advise resection or transplantation.

Most patients cannot undergo resection due to the extensive nature of the disease and the risk of precipitating liver failure because of underlying cirrhosis. Only a small subgroup is considered for transplantation. However, the outcome after liver transplantation is poor for patients with advanced stage hepatomas because of recurrence of cancer. Patients with advanced stage cancer are considered for palliative treatment with either chemoembolization, cryosurgery, or radiofrequency thermal ablation.

(3) Metastatic Liver Cancer. Patients with widespread tumor that has metastasized (spread) beyond the confines of the liver are not candidates for surgery, transplantation, cryotherapy, or chemoembolization. They are evaluated only for standard chemotherapy.

Hepatic Resection. Surgeons achieve the best results in the treatment of hepatoma when they perform a liver resection to surgically remove a solitary tumor (less than five centimeters) in a patient with a noncirrhotic liver. These patients may be cured of their cancer and usually enjoy long-term survival.

However, this represents an uncommon clinical scenario when it comes to hepatoma in patients with hepatitis B. As I have already mentioned, at least 50 percent of people with hepatitis B who develop a liver cancer have cirrhosis and a disease duration of hepatitis B for greater than 30 years.

> *My brother was diagnosed with hepatitis B. Two weeks later, they found liver cancer, and a week after that he was dead. It was devastating.*
>
> *Somewhere in my mother's past, she was told she had hepatitis B and not to worry. Were we infected at birth? We'll never know. But two of my mother's sisters tested positive and my grandfather died when I was 14 of some kind of "stomach trouble."*
>
> *The world does not understand what hepatitis B can do to you.*
>
> *Polly*

Unfortunately, cirrhosis precludes a successful resection because resections for hepatoma usually require removing 25 to 75 percent of the liver tissue. A normal liver can tolerate a large resection since regeneration is rapid (usually within 12 weeks), and the remaining liver cells are functioning normally. That's not the case when a person has cirrhosis and hepatitis B; the remaining liver cannot effectively regenerate, and its function is severely impaired. When a surgeon performs a large resection on a cirrhotic patient, the operation may lead to liver failure. For these reasons liver resections are usually restricted to patients without cirrhosis or to those cirrhotic patients who have no evidence of clinical or biochemical deterioration in liver function or portal hypertension.

Transplantation. Results from a number of centers agree. Cirrhotic patients with solitary liver cancers, small in size (less than five centimeters in diameter) or up to three tumors (all less than three centimeters in diameter), should be considered for transplantation.

Successful transplantation may also be performed on patients with multiple tumor nodules (all less than two centimeters) that are restricted to one hepatic lobe with no evidence of invasion of blood vessels. Although these two groups of patients can expect long-term, tumor-free survival, those with advanced stages of hepatoma or metastatic disease almost uniformly experience early post-transplant recurrence of tumor and death from metastatic disease. Transplantation is not indicated for the latter patients.

Even for hepatomas in favorable stages, time can run out. Most of the data that deals with successful transplants for hepatoma come from an era of relatively greater donor liver availability. That situation no longer exists in this country. The U.S. waiting list for liver transplantation continues to expand. As of December 2000, over 16,000 patients were on the list, but only about 4,500 liver transplants are performed annually.

Patients with hepatoma are at a distinct disadvantage as they wait for a liver. The tumor will grow with time, spread to adjacent areas of the liver, invade blood vessels, and prevent the patient from continuing as a transplant candidate. In the future, patients with hepatoma will need to be considered for living-donor liver transplantation (see Chapter 9).

Given current statistics, I project that by the year 2015 the U.S. waiting list will contain 30,000 to 45,000 patients. Nearly three-quarters of these patients will have either hepatitis B or C, and a sizeable number of them may develop hepatoma while waiting for a donor liver.

Chemoembolization. This procedure does not cure cancer. However, it can help destroy local tumors, reduce the tumor mass, provide significant relief, or in the case of a solitary tumor, keep the tumor from spreading outside the liver until a donor liver becomes available.

> *The room was kept very cold—for the machine, they said. The doctor cut the artery in my right leg just below my groin. They put a clamp around it, and a technician threaded a narrow, thin catheter up through the artery into my liver. I watched it on a TV screen.*
>
> *He maneuvered the catheter into capillaries feeding the hepatoma. I could see it was there. Then they mixed up a potent cancer drug and injected it for about ten minutes. The hope is that none of the poison will escape so you won't have side effects.*
>
> *I didn't have any nausea, and I didn't lose my hair. Now I have an MRI every six months. It's been two years, and the scar tissue is less each time.*
>
> *Owen*

The technique involves placing a catheter through a vessel in the groin (the femoral artery) and advancing it into the liver's main artery (the hepatic artery). Then a special form of chemotherapy is infused through the catheter into the artery feeding the tumor. Both normal and hepatoma cells take up the chemotherapy, but cancer cells do not excrete it. Because cancer cells retain the chemotherapy for a prolonged time, they are destroyed.

In the absence of resection or transplantation, chemoembolization is not curative, and the patient should understand that the tumor will probably recur. Nonetheless, chemoembolization of the tumor has been associated with prolonged survival and reduced symptoms of pain and weight loss. In transplant candidates, chemoembolization may sustain the patient until successful transplantation can take place.

High-Frequency Radio Waves (Radiofrequency Tumor Ablation). This treatment of hepatoma remains under study. The technique involves CT-guided puncture of the hepatoma and positioning the prongs of a special instrument within the tumor mass. High-frequency radio waves (near the microwave limit) generated within the tumor mass destroy the tumor. Overall effectiveness and clinical outcome of this treatment for hepatoma remain to be defined.

Alcohol Injection, Cryosurgery. These two approaches are also limited to hepatomas that cannot be resected or transplanted. The goal of these treatments is to reduce tumor size and relieve painful symptoms.

Alcohol injection is done with the guidance of a CT scan to ensure proper placement of the treatment catheter within the tumor. Absolute alcohol dehydrates the tissues, causing the immediate death of cells, and starts a clotting process within the tumor that destroys it.

Cryosurgery involves the use of a flexible fiberoptic instrument (laparoscopy) with the guidance of an ultrasound probe to properly position the cryosurgical instrument within the tumor. When the probe is positioned, the tumor cells are destroyed by freezing.

Chemotherapy. Hepatoma is one of the most resistant tumors to both radiation and chemotherapy. Early experience with external beam radiation suggested that doses of radiation required for effective anti-tumor activity exceeded safety standards. In addition, clinical experience with radiation therapy of hepatomas was uniformly dismal and disappointing. For this reason, radiation is employed only rarely in the treatment of these tumors. Some evidence suggests that chemotherapy can be partially effective in reducing tumor burden and relieving symptoms.

Summary

Primary liver cancer is an extremely serious, life-threatening complication of chronic hepatitis B. It occurs mainly in patients with advanced disease and cirrhosis but also in noncirrhotic patients who acquired hepatitis B vertically from an infected mother at the time of delivery. Screening of these two populations, using alpha-fetoprotein and ultrasonography, is recommended. Hepatitis B patients with bridging fibrosis or cirrhosis should be aware of the danger of liver cancer, undergo screening by their physician, and know the warning signs.

Early hepatoma is treatable, but most patients with large tumors or multiple tumors cannot be treated by liver resection or transplantation. Cirrhotic patients with solitary and small hepatomas should be considered for early liver transplantation and possibly living-donor transplantation. A number of new approaches can reduce, but not cure, inoperable tumors: chemoembolization, radiofrequency thermal ablation, alcohol ablation, cryosurgery, and systemic chemotherapy.

Liver cancer is an increasingly important issue for hepatitis B patients, families, physicians, surgeons, transplant programs, and the health care system in general. We in the medical community know that we sorely need new ideas and new treatments.

The first wealth is health.

Emerson

11

HIV/AIDS,
HEPATITIS C, AND
DELTA CO-INFECTION:
Triple Trouble

In 1996 the doctors took me off AZT and put me on triple combination drug therapy. My T-cells went up, and my viral load went down. The nurse said they could probably keep me alive for a long time if I stayed off drugs and cocaine.

Meanwhile, two friends, who also had AIDS, killed themselves. The loneliness, deaths, and suicides were too much. Then I found out I had hepatitis C in August. I was tired all the time, so they tested me—and the tests came back reactive for hepatitis B and C.

I cried. I started reading about hepatitis, and none of it looked good. Another virus. Now I have three viruses in my body.

Jay

THIS CHAPTER DISCUSSES several different types of viral co-infections: HIV, hepatitis C, and hepatitis D (Delta). If you are battling hepatitis B, it can be devastating to discover that you have another viral infection, HIV/AIDS. Conversely, if you have been diagnosed with HIV/AIDS, it is extremely difficult to find out that you also have hepatitis B. Perhaps you are co-infected with hepatitis C or hepatitis D, Delta. It is possible, although unlikely, that you could be infected with three or four viruses simultaneously.

You know from personal experience what it means to live with one dangerous virus and now you have to face co-infection. Nothing can prepare you for the shock. Once again, you go through the cycle of fear, anger, and denial

Until a few years ago, doctors did not focus on treating hepatitis B in people with AIDS because patients with AIDS had limited years to live. Also, interferon treatment affected the immune system, which was already impaired by AIDS. Now, however, the introduction of new highly active AIDS drugs (HAART therapy) has produced a growing number of HIV-infected patients with strengthened immune systems who are enjoying longer life spans. With this hopeful and encouraging development, treatment of hepatitis B in patients with HIV infection becomes a greater concern.

Co-infection with hepatitis C or Delta alters your prognosis and raises treatment issues. Patients co-infected with hepatitis C and Delta tend to have more aggressive liver disease with a greater likelihood of progression to cirrhosis and the need for a liver transplant. Also, the risk of cancer increases in patients co-infected with hepatitis C. Patients with Delta co-infection are less likely to respond to therapy with either interferon or lamivudine. When dealing with hepatitis B and C co-infection, the doctor must assess and determine the dominant agent and tailor treatment to the dominant virus.

In this chapter, I will discuss the following topics:

- Overview of HIV Co-Infection
  What Is HIV/AIDS?
  Testing Problems
  Population Trends
- Current Treatment of HIV Infection
  Highly Active Anti-Retroviral Therapies (HAART)
- Complications of HAART Therapy
  Effect of Hepatitis B Infection on HIV
  Effect of HIV Infection on Hepatitis B
- Does HIV Co-Infection Affect the Rate of Progression of Liver Disease?

- Antiviral Therapy of Hepatitis B for People Co-Infected with HIV
    Are New Treatments on the Horizon for Co-Infected Patients?
- Co-Infection with Hepatitis C
- Co-Infection with Hepatitis D (Delta)
- Liver Transplantation
    Transplantation before HAART
    Transplantation after HAART
- Summary

Overview of HIV Co-Infection

What IS HIV/AIDS? The human immunodeficiency virus (HIV) destroys the immune system that helps the body fight illness and infection. HIV infects lymphocytes, the main immune cells in the body, and causes acquired immunodeficiency syndrome (AIDS). Severe damage to the immune system results in susceptibility to a wide array of infections and malignancy (cancer).

According to the Centers for Disease Control and Prevention (CDC) December 1997 figures, an estimated 650,000 to 900,000 people are living with HIV/AIDS in the United States—about 0.3 percent of the population. Worldwide, the estimated number of people living with HIV/AIDS is 30.6 million.

Many people with AIDS are also infected with the hepatitis B virus (HBV) because some behaviors that transmit AIDS also transmit hepatitis B (such as sexual contact; sharing intravenous drug needles; and receiving blood transfusions, organ transplants, or hemophilia treatment before tests screened the nation's blood supply). When AIDS patients are infected with both HIV and HBV, it is called an HIV/HBV co-infection.

In my experience, HIV treatment clinics diagnose most cases of HIV/HBV co-infection because symptoms relating to HIV usually emerge before those of hepatitis B. In fact, I have personally diagnosed unsuspected HIV in only a handful of patients with chronic hepatitis B, despite years of experience in our hepatology clinics. Even so, we recommend routine testing for HIV in patients with chronic hepatitis B.

I had my first boyfriend at 19. He didn't know it, but he was HIV positive. No one had heard of HIV at the time so there were no precautions for it. Then we began to hear about the virus.

When I had one year of college left, I felt it was my obligation to get tested. It was a horrible time. Hysteria surrounded HIV. I did test positive, and it was horrendous, traumatic. At 21, I thought I'd die sooner, rather than later.

I had been vaccinated for hepatitis B at 19, but when I was 25, my liver enzymes started to go up. I remember showering and looking at my ankle and thinking it looked yellow. The enzymes went pretty high, but the doctors thought it was due to a common side effect of the HIV drugs. Finally, I went to another doctor who tested for HBV. I found out I was co-infected with chronic hepatitis B.

I probably had half an immune system when I got vaccinated so maybe that's why it didn't work for me. I was pretty depressed because I saw the diagnosis of hepatitis B as an indication that the HIV was getting worse, that my immune system was declining. Hepatitis B was more like another symptom that fell under the umbrella of HIV—like another opportunistic infection is how I saw it.

Joel

Testing Problems. How many people with HIV are also infected with hepatitis B? The prevalence of hepatitis B in patients with HIV varies with the population studied and with the type of testing used to detect HBV. For example, HBV DNA testing may detect virus even in patients who test negative for hepatitis B surface antigen. Studies using surface antigen testing may, therefore, underestimate the prevalence of HBV in the HIV population. Unfortunately, nearly all prevalence data have relied on data from surface antigen or antibody testing, not on the measurement of HBV DNA (see Chapter 2 for a discussion of these different types of tests).

Population Trends. In one study, 94 pediatric AIDS patients (ages 12 to 20) were examined for markers of active hepatitis B or prior immunization (mainly by vaccination). Nineteen percent were co-infected with hepatitis B (13 percent of the females and 30 percent of the males), 16 percent had been immunized, and 65 percent were not immune and susceptible to infection with HBV. A retrospective study of 394 adults with HIV infection initiating HAART treatment identified a 7 percent prevalence of active chronic hepatitis B.

I was married for 25 years and had four children. I got a divorce. I knew I was gay, and I couldn't live a lie anymore. Then I started acting out sexually.

In 1980, I went to the doctor because I was jaundiced. "There's not much to do but suffer through it," he said. He hadn't heard of hepatitis B—didn't have a clue.

Nine years later, I was diagnosed with HIV, and three years after that I had a relapse of the hepatitis. A biopsy showed I had some cirrhosis—mild, not severe.

HIV is scarier than chronic hepatitis because I heard such horror stories about HIV. I haven't experienced an immune deficiency problem, which is very fortunate. I don't talk about hepatitis B. I will admit that I'm practically celibate at this stage of the game.

Carl

Co-infection with hepatitis B is more likely in patients with HIV due to similar transmission routes, such as intravenous drug abuse or male homosexuality. Additional risk factors for hepatitis B were assessed in a study of 328 unvaccinated male homosexuals with HIV, 41 percent of whom had markers for exposure to hepatitis B or had active hepatitis B. The risk of infection with hepatitis B was related to a history of other sexually transmitted diseases, particularly those that cause ulcers of the genitals (e.g., herpes, gonococcal, or syphilitic infections). Other risk factors included injection drug use, having a sexual partner with HIV/AIDS, and a history of high-level sexual promiscuity (more than 50 partners).

Resource: For information on co-infection with HIV and HBV, access the Website: www.hivandhepatitis.com

Current Treatment of HIV Infection

HIV is an RNA virus acquired by blood-borne routes or sexual activity. The virus, first identified in 1983 as the cause of AIDS, was given the name human T-cell lymphotropic virus type III (HTLV-III) in the United States because of its known association with lymphocytes. HIV infects the body's immune cells (lymphocytes), which then become dysfunctional, nonfunctional, or die, thus severely impairing the body's immune system. Before current effective anti-HIV therapy, most patients succumbed to either the ravages of infectious disease or malignancy.

I have post-traumatic stress disorder. My best friend died of AIDS, and I remember feeling numb, confused. This existence is so random, uncaring. I couldn't make sense of what was happening around me.

I started a support group for people in their 20s who were HIV positive. I found strength in numbers and comraderie. But every so often, someone wouldn't show up—and we'd find out they died.

Bill

Highly Active Anti-Retroviral Therapies (HAART). Two classes of drugs, reverse transcriptase inhibitors and protease inhibitors, have dramatically altered the course of HIV infection. Today, most patients with HIV are treated with a combination of three to four drugs, and they experience significant improvement.

How effective are these highly active anti-retroviral therapies (HAART)? Steven C. Johnson, M.D., Associate Professor of Medicine and Director of the University Hospital HIV/AIDS Clinical Program, University of Colorado Health Sciences Center, reviewed outcomes over a three-year period.[1] From 1995 through 1997 the percentage of AIDS patients treated with HAART increased from less than 10 percent to over 80 percent. The rate of hospitalization fell from 6.4 to 1.1 inpatient days per patient-year. Decreases in days of hospitalization resulted in significant cost reductions. The incidence of the three major opportunistic infections (infections that develop only because of the patient's immune deficiency)—pneumocystis pneumonia, mycobacterium avium complex disease, and cytomegalovirus retinitis (CMV)—decreased dramatically. Death from opportunistic infection or advanced HIV declined markedly from 15 percent of the clinic population in 1994 to 2 percent in 1998.

Hepatitis and end-stage liver disease, however, emerged as an important cause of sickness and death in this population. In 1995 hepatitis and liver disease accounted for only 4 percent of deaths, but two years later the number rose to 14 percent!

Resources: For more information about the current treatment for HIV/AIDS, contact the following hotlines and information services:

CDC National HIV/AIDS Hotline: 1-800-342-2437 (English); 1-800-344-7432 (Spanish); 1-800-243-7889 (TDD)

CDC National Sexually Transmitted Diseases (STD) Hotline: 1-800-227-8922

CDC Website: www.cdc.gov

Complications of HAART Therapy

Effect of Hepatitis B Infection on HIV. Co-infection with hepatitis B can certainly complicate the treatment and clinical course of HIV infection. Currently, the Federal Drug Administration has licensed more than 13 drugs for treatment of HIV in the United States. Nearly all of these medications, but in particular the protease inhibitors, are metabolized in some way by the liver.

As liver disease due to hepatitis B progresses from hepatitis to cirrhosis, the liver is less able to metabolize these compounds. Changes in liver function may make it necessary to change the drugs used and the doses of individual drugs. In addition, the anti–HIV drugs may be toxic to the liver. Instances of liver enzyme elevations, jaundice, and even fatal cases of severe liver toxicity from anti–HIV medications have occurred.

A recent study examined the development of abnormal liver tests after starting 394 HIV patients on HAART treatment. Seven percent were co-infected with hepatitis B and 14 percent had hepatitis C. The risk of developing abnormal liver tests was greater in HIV patients who had chronic hepatitis (37 percent vs. 12 percent in HIV patients without either HBV or HCV).

My doctor said there was a drug called interferon for hepatitis B, but because I was HIV positive, it wouldn't work—so I changed doctors. The next doctor put me on interferon, and I responded so he upped me to six million units. I took it after work, and by bedtime I slept it off. My enzymes went back down. I was very happy, and I did that for a couple of years.

About that time, protease inhibitors came out. I held out for a drug called Crixvan®. It was hard to take, but I was determined. My T-cells doubled in a month and started creeping up. It was the first time in ten years I saw such a dramatic improvement. After spending ten years fighting for your life, suddenly you've got it!

Then, a year after the HIV drugs worked, the HBV broke through. My liver enzymes went up. I think there's a connection. A giant monster called HIV was at my shoulder, ready to pounce on me. I slew the monster. Then a little gnat called HBV suddenly rose in importance. I'm living longer, and suddenly what seemed small potatoes became a primary concern. Equally frustrating was that if the liver enzymes got too high, I'd have to stop the HIV drugs.

Doug

One additional fear is that HAART medications may accelerate the progression of hepatitis B to cirrhosis in patients with active hepatitis B (positive hepatitis B surface antigen) and therefore compromise the effectiveness of therapy against HIV. In addition, several reports have suggested that patients with hepatitis B surface antibody (who were previously thought to be cleared of hepatitis B) activated hepatitis B under HAART. The latter observation is of particular importance for two reasons. First, as many as 30 to 70 percent of HIV-infected patients have antibodies, indicating prior exposure to hepatitis B and the potential for reactivation under HAART. Second, all HIV patients with liver disease attributed to progressive hepatitis C under HAART should be examined for evidence of activation of hepatitis B (blood should be tested for HBsAg, HBeAg, HBV DNA).

Effect of HIV Infection on Hepatitis B. As described in preceding chapters, a chronic hepatitis B patient's own immune system can injure the liver as the immune system tries to destroy infected liver cells (immune-mediated injury). In contrast, in the post-transplant setting, viral levels are very high due to the use of immunosuppressive medications, and the virus itself destroys liver cells. Thus, HIV infection, which destroys components of the immune response, may either slow or accelerate liver disease due to hepatitis B.

> *I was on a research program with interferon. I had a terrible time tolerating it. They kept reducing my dosage. I had extreme exhaustion; I couldn't function. The cure was worse than the disease.*
>
> *Finally, I had to terminate with their approval. My system said no thanks. Live with what you've got. What I didn't know at the time was that I had HIV.*
>
> Fred

In one of the best-designed studies, Colin and colleagues examined the influence of HIV infection on chronic hepatitis B. Patients who previously received therapy for hepatitis B were excluded, and none of the HIV-infected patients had received lamivudine. In their series, 67 patients with chronic hepatitis B were compared to 65 patients co-infected with HBV and HIV. Eighteen of the 65 HIV-infected patients were taking zidovudine monotherapy and three were taking combination zidovudine plus dideoxycytidine. None of the patients had either hepatitis C or Delta infection.

Co-infected patients had lower ALT levels, lower serum albumin, and higher serum levels of HBV DNA. Despite the lower level ALT and similar scores for inflammation on liver biopsy, co-infected patients were more likely to have cirrhosis. Co-infected patients had a greater risk for cirrhosis even after correction by sophisticated statistical analysis for the effects of age and alcohol use. One could conclude that progressive liver injury leading to cirrhosis may occur in co-infected patients even when the ALT is relatively low.

An earlier study in 1987, by Krogsgaard, compared 25 patients with chronic hepatitis B to eight co-infected patients. Co-infected patients were less likely to spontaneously clear HBV DNA and e antigen and had lower ALT levels.

These results are consistent with two theories about how liver injury is caused by hepatitis B: immune-mediated injury and direct toxic effect on cells by the virus (cytotoxicity). In HIV infection the immune response is blunted, the immune-mediated injury triggered by infection with hepatitis B is suppressed, and the ALT is relatively lower. On the other hand, the immune deficiency caused by HIV also favors replication of the hepatitis B virus and lowers the likelihood for spontaneous clearance of HBV. Enhanced replication results in increased blood levels of HBV DNA and an increased risk for the direct cytotoxicity of the hepatitis B virus on liver cells. However, larger controlled trials would be required to verify that progression to cirrhosis is more rapid in co-infected patients. If true, this finding would suggest a greater role for viral replication than for immune-mediated mechanisms in liver injury and fibrosis.

HIV is like a fire burning. You need a big bucket of water to put it out. You need powerful meds when it's raging, then less "water" to keep it down. Today I take a combo twice a day—a cocktail light. The regimens are getting easier.

For four years, I've had pretty good blood tests on the HIV front. On the HBV front, I discovered adefovir: 120 milligrams, a really high dose. It drove the HBV viral load down to nothing.

Here's the problem with experimental drugs—they're experimental. I was thrilled and thought I'd broken the odds again, but then I had to keep lowering the dose because it was affecting my kidneys. Ultimately, it was not approved for HIV because of this, but the dosage for HBV now is 10 milligrams a day.

My doctor said, "Stop. You don't want to see kidney damage because drugs are coming down the road that will have activity for HBV."

Eric

Does HIV Co-Infection Affect the Rate of Progression of Liver Disease?

The CDC has reported that the percentage of HIV patients with death due to liver disease steadily increased between 1987 to 1997. According to data from the U.S. National Vital Statistics System, the percent of death certificates listing "sequelae (consequences) of chronic liver disease" increased from 1.3 percent in 1987, 2.2 percent in 1995, to 3.5 percent in 1997.

Further analysis of death certificates indicated that liver disease caused, contributed, or was secondarily involved in approximately 10 percent of all deaths in 1997. Patients dying with a diagnosis of chronic hepatitis C increased from 0.9 percent in 1995 to 2.3 percent in 1997 (tests for hepatitis C were not available until 1990). Patients dying with a diagnosis of chronic hepatitis B increased from 0.5 percent in 1987, 0.8 percent in 1995, to 1.3 percent in 1997.

The observed increase in deaths related to "sequelae of chronic liver disease" exceeded the expected frequency by 46 percent. It is not known whether the increase in mortality rate was due to use of HAART medications, increased activity of hepatitis viruses, or reflected the natural progression of hepatitis B and C occurring in HIV patients who now live longer.

Antiviral Therapy of Hepatitis B for People Co-Infected with HIV

The published literature regarding antiviral therapy of co-infected patients is limited, and nearly all reports represent observational or anecdotal experience. Experience with interferon-alfa, in reports of studies conducted before HAART, was abysmal with inhibition of HBV viral replication in less than 8 percent of cases. There was no benefit of therapy in the only controlled trial of interferon alfa (reported in 1995) in a male homosexual population with co-infection. For these reasons, interferon treatment has not been recommended in co-infected patients.

The success of HAART and the development of pegylated interferons now have rekindled interest in interferon-based treatment of co-infected patients. I anticipate that results of current clinical trials will indicate improved results with interferon monotherapy or interferon in combination with other antivirals (ribavirin, lamivudine, entecavir, or adefovir).

> *I'm depressed about having hepatitis B, but I know from our experience with AIDS that we can overcome. It sounds corny, but I know there's hope. And I keep close tabs on drug development.*
>
> *Lee*

Lamivudine has been the mainstay of antiviral therapy for hepatitis B in co-infected patients. In fact, the observation that HIV/HBV co-infected patients had suppression of HBV DNA during lamivudine treatment for HIV prompted the general use of lamivudine in patients infected solely with chronic hepatitis B.

One recent report examined the long-term effects of lamivudine on 66 co-infected patients who were receiving 150 milligrams twice daily (300 mg/d) as treatment for their HIV infection. Prior to treatment all of the patients had detectable HBV DNA in blood. Within two months of treatment, 86.4 percent became HBV DNA negative, but the majority of treated patients developed resistance to lamivudine over time. By the second year of therapy, 53 percent had broken through and become HBV DNA positive (mostly due to emergence of YMDD mutations, see Chapter 8).

The authors estimated the risk of breakthrough at 20 percent per year, suggesting that after five years of treatment nearly all co-infected patients would develop lamivudine resistance. The effect of these virologic events on liver injury and disease progression in co-infected patients is unknown. However, this experience is prompting many investigators to initiate trials of combination therapy (lamivudine plus adefovir is one promising combination).

Are New Treatments on the Horizon for Co-Infected Patients?
The future holds genuine promise for effective future therapies for co-infected patients. HAART has changed the landscape. Therapies once considered ineffective in co-infected patients, such as interferon alfa,

may re-emerge as effective treatment options. The effectiveness of interferon has been enhanced by the development of sustained, long-acting pegylated interferons (modification of the parent molecules with polyethylene glycol polymers), and improved rates of viral clearance should be expected.

> *The gay community sparked a new philosophy of a patient's role in his health care. People learned to tell scientists and doctors what they wanted. It was a unique time to be alive.*
>
> *I felt part of a larger group, part of a cause. I had a purpose, a mission. Life wasn't about a great first job or about buying things. Life was about getting drugs, medicines, and information and making an impact on the world around you.*
>
> *Ray*

Interestingly, the combination of interferon plus ribavirin, which has dramatically improved rates of response in patients with hepatitis C, may also be effective in chronic hepatitis B. Additional trials are examining the combination of interferon with lamivudine, and other nucleoside analogues.

Other nucleoside analogues are also promising. Entecavir is currently in clinical trials and may be 100 to 1000 times more potent than lamivudine. Current results with adefovir dipivoxil are promising and indicate that this therapy may be highly effective in patients with YMDD mutation. The latter finding has generated interest in using adefovir in combination with either lamivudine or entecavir (see Chapters 8 and 13). Two additional emerging therapies include DAPD and L-FMAU. Your doctor may be able to tell you if you are a candidate for participating in trials of any of these therapies.

Resources: For more information about treatment and trials, contact the following:
1. AIDS Treatment Information Service (ATIS): 1-800-448-0440
2. Project Inform: 1-800-822-7422
3. AIDS Clinical Trials Information Service: 1-800-TRIALS-A
4. www.hivandhepatitis.com

Co-Infection with Hepatitis C

I have hepatitis C and B—but I feel worse about B for some reason. I associate it with dirt, uncleanliness or something. I think I compare it to AIDS. I don't want hepatitis B. It scares me.

When I go to the dentist, instead of putting on one pair of latex gloves, they always double-glove. And sometimes when I have the inclination to give someone a hug, they just stand there. Now I wait for them to give me a hug first.

Naomi

The worst thing for me is the fatigue. Although everyone with hepatitis seems to suffer to some degree, my experience has been extreme. My doctor thinks that maybe because I have two viruses, B and C, my body fights twice as hard and causes me to be increasingly more tired.

Mel

Co-infection with hepatitis B and C, each of which independently damages the liver, results in greater liver damage and more rapid progression to cirrhosis. Current estimates suggest that 10 to 15 percent of patients with chronic hepatitis B are co-infected with hepatitis C. In addition, "hidden" infection with hepatitis B (hepatitis B surface antigen negative) may occur in up to 33 percent of patients with chronic hepatitis C. Two-thirds of the latter patients have isolated hepatitis B core antibody, and one-third lack all serologic markers for hepatitis B but have positive HBV DNA. Although co-infection may suppress rates of viral replication, and levels of HBV DNA or HCV RNA may be relatively lower, liver damage is increased.

A recent case-control study confirmed the reciprocal relationship between inhibition of viral replication and liver damage. Co-infected patients, despite lower viral replication, were more likely to have either moderate to severe chronic hepatitis or cirrhosis. Co-infected patients may also have a greater risk of developing hepatocellular carcinoma, liver cancer (see Chapter 10).

In general, therapy is recommended for co-infected patients. Doctors often try to determine which of the two viruses dominate the other (in terms of contributing to the liver injury) in order to choose therapy. This decision is often based upon the tests for hepatitis B. The patient with positive HBV DNA and hepatitis B e antigen may have dominant hepatitis B and warrant lamivudine or daily interferon in relatively high doses for four to six months. The patient who is negative for HBV DNA and hepatitis B e antigen may have dominant hepatitis C and warrant combination interferon plus ribavirin for up to one year.

With me, the C is the active virus and the B is apparently rather inert. I was so tired and irritable, I had to quit night school—and my goal was to finish college before my kids. When I tried to go back, there was no brain left. I had migraines, joint pain, arthritis.

I read that if you have B as well, the hepatitis is worse so I decided to try treatment. I made my husband promise not to leave me if I went on interferon. The first night, my husband and I sat on the couch and waited for the side effects. We both fell asleep.

When I woke up, I had no joint pain. It's been eight months, and I feel better on interferon. My labs are good. The C is undetectable.

Ina

My son, a hemophiliac, tested positive for hepatitis B at age one. He was also diagnosed with hepatitis C, although at that time they called it non-A/non-B hepatitis. He got hepatitis from clotting factor they gave him to stop the bleeds. Today they heat the clotting factor to kill viruses.

He's 19 now and more concerned about being contagious with the hepatitis B in regard to his social life. His doctor started him on six months of combo therapy for the C, but with daily doses of interferon to hit the B hard. In July he tested negative for the first time ever for hepatitis B surface antigens. And he tested less than 200 for a hepatitis C viral load after a six-month treatment of daily interferon and ribavirin!

Sophie

Recent evidence suggests that ribavirin may also be effective against hepatitis B. This observation, coupled with the emergence of pegylated interferons, suggests that the best future therapy for co-infected patients may be the combination of pegylated interferon with ribavirin. Regardless of choice of therapy, effectiveness must be determined with PCR tests to measure both HBV DNA and HCV RNA (see Chapter 2). Subsequent treatment should be tailored to the outcome of the first course.

In clinical practice, liver biopsy does not help to determine the dominance of one infection over the other because the histologic (cell) changes with hepatitis B and C are similar. Research tests (including immunohistochemical examination and molecular studies of biopsy material) may be able to distinguish the dominant infection, but their clinical usefulness is not defined.

> *I didn't have a clue I was sick until I had a bleed. I was in the hospital eight or nine days. When the tests came back, they were positive for hepatitis B and C. My biopsy showed I only had 25 percent liver function. I had cirrhosis so bad, the doctor said I was a candidate for a transplant. I had active hepatitis C and inactive hepatitis B. The fear was that after the transplant, because of the immunosuppressive drugs and the surgery, the B could flare up.*
>
> *Juliet*

Resource: For more information on hepatitis C, contact the organizations listed in the Resources section at the end of this book and the Hep C Connection, 1177 Grant St., Suite 200, Denver, CO 80203. Phone: 303-860-0800. Hep C Hotline: 1-800-522-HEPC. Email: info@hepc-connection.org. Website: www.hepc-connection.org
Resource: Everson, Gregory T., M.D., and Hedy Weinberg. *Living with Hepatitis C: A Survivor's Guide.* Long Island City: Hatherleigh Press, 1999 (2nd edition), 2001 (3rd edition).

Co-Infection with Hepatitis D (Delta)

Delta co-infection is relatively rare in U.S. patients and is diminishing in importance in Southern Europe due to the increasing use of universal vaccination against hepatitis B. Risk factors for acquiring Delta infection are similar to the risks of acquiring hepatitis B.

> *Thirty years ago, I was yellow and peeing black. They didn't have a name for it except infectious serum hepatitis. I was doing a lot of hard drugs. God saved me then, but I was stupid. I didn't get clean until 1977—and now I'm crispy clean and doing the middle class thing.*
>
> *Almost 20 years later, my liver enzymes were high. I had a biopsy— end-stage cirrhosis. I needed a transplant. It was the first time I heard the name chronic hepatitis B. The test results for D took six more weeks.*

Delta was not a real important thing to me. I only knew that it was very rare and manifested itself in Mediterranean cultures. I don't think it made me sicker, but I don't know. The doctors said there was some evidence that Delta might help me do better after the transplant. But another doctor wouldn't respond when I told him that.

Andrew

Delta virus is a defective RNA virus that requires the hepatitis B surface antigen to complete its replication. For this reason, Delta infection only occurs in the setting of hepatitis B infection (positive hepatitis B surface antigen). Interestingly, Delta suppresses the replication of hepatitis B, and patients with chronic Delta hepatitis typically test negative for e antigen and HBV DNA and positive for e antibody.

The infection is diagnosed by testing for specific antibody (anti-HDV) and confirmed by the presence of HDV RNA in the blood or HDV antigen in the liver. Chronic Delta infection has been associated with more aggressive hepatitis and a greater likelihood of developing cirrhosis. Reports vary but suggest that 30 to 70 percent of infected individuals will develop cirrhosis.

The treatment of Delta is directed at the underlying hepatitis B infection. One randomized controlled trial studied 42 patients with chronic hepatitis D. Patients received either interferon-alfa-2a, 9 million units three times a week (9 MU tiw) for 48 weeks; 3 million units three times a week (3 MU tiw) for 48 weeks; or no treatment.

On treatment, 50 percent of those receiving the 9 MU dose had a complete response with normalization of ALT and clearance of HDV RNA. However, relapse of Delta infection occurred universally; no patient had a sustained clearance of the Delta virus. Relapse occurred even after prolonged periods of two to six months of testing negative for the virus. Despite the inability to clear the virus, many patients experienced prolonged normalization of ALT levels, even though they had a relapse of viral infection. One patient with chronic Delta, who had relapsed after standard courses of therapy, was given interferon-alfa-2b (5 MU qd) every day for 12 years and demonstrated clearance of viral infection, normalization of ALT, and histological resolution of cirrhosis.

One could conclude from this information that it is difficult to eradicate established chronic Delta infection using interferon in hepatitis B patients who are negative for e antigen and HBV DNA. However, prolonged therapy may lead to viral clearance and appears to have positive effects on the liver disease.

The safety and efficacy of lamivudine in hepatitis B led investigators to examine its usefulness in chronic Delta infection. Five patients were given lamivudine, 100 milligrams a day for 12 months. All remained positive for hepatitis B surface antigen and HDV RNA throughout the course of treatment. Neither serum ALT nor liver histology improved.

Results with the combination of interferon plus lamivudine have been equally disappointing. Thus, lamivudine would seem to have no role in the treatment of chronic Delta hepatitis. Lamivudine might still be considered for candidates for liver transplantation because lamivudine does significantly suppress HBV DNA, even in patients with Delta, and might reduce the risk of the recurrence of HDV/HBV co-infection after liver transplantation.

Liver Transplantation

Patients co-infected with HBV/HCV, HBV/HDV, or HBV/HCV/HDV are considered candidates for liver transplantation using the same criteria established for isolated HBV. Transplantation for patients co-infected with HIV is controversial and there are only limited reports from a few centers.

Transplantation before HAART. Before HAART physicians refused to consider HIV-infected patients for liver transplantation for the following reasons: (1) The immunosuppressive medications used after transplantation to prevent rejection of the donor liver would have further compromised the HIV-induced immune deficiency and increased the risk of serious life-threatening infection or malignancy. (2) HIV patients typically had ongoing infections, malignancies, or other illnesses that prohibited transplantation. (3) HIV patients would likely have died of HIV-related complications despite liver transplantation, thereby wasting a donor liver.

Anecdotal reports of liver transplantation in HIV-infected patients before the era of HAART therapy indicated that HIV patients continued to have HIV after the transplant. They experienced a predictable downhill course. Therefore, many transplant centers disqualified HIV patients from receiving liver transplants. Current Medicare guidelines indicate that HIV is an absolute contraindication to liver transplantation.

I'm really worried. If I get cirrhosis, they won't give me a transplant because I have AIDS. That will be it. The end. No options.

The only thing that keeps me going is God.

Reuben

Transplantation after HAART. HAART therapy may make liver transplantation an option for HIV-infected patients. HAART therapy has been so effective that the projected life span for an HIV-infected individual now extends from less than five years to more than 20 years. Patients co-infected with HIV/HBV may remain stable in terms of the complications of their immune deficiency only to experience significant liver disease, liver failure, and the need for liver transplantation.

At the University of Colorado Health Sciences Center, deaths of HIV-infected patients in 1997 were nearly as often due to hepatitis and end-stage liver disease as to opportunistic infections or malignancy. In fact, deaths due to liver disease surpassed deaths due to advanced HIV, which includes AIDS wasting syndrome and dementia. Although many centers performing liver transplants now are revisiting the question, there is still great reluctance to perform liver transplants in HIV patients.

Summary

We are just beginning to address the growing problem of co-infection with multiple viruses. As patients with HIV/AIDS live decades longer due to new treatments, many of them will have to deal with hepatitis B treatment decisions. These are complicated issues because HIV/AIDS therapies affect the liver, and hepatitis B therapies affect the immune system.

My hope is that new studies, advances in drug therapy, and controlled research projects will yield more information about all of these viruses. Then physicians and patients can work together to make thoughtful plans for treatment and to offer more options to patients affected by HIV/AIDS, hepatitis B, C, and Delta.

A journey of a thousand miles must begin with a single step.

Lao-tzu

Reference

[1] S. Johnson, A. Hageman, H. Wing, M. Grodesky, N. Bathurst, P. Romfh, W. Williams. Effect of Antiretroviral Therapy on Clinical Outcomes and Cost in a University-Based HIV/AIDS Program: 1995-1997. Abstract 42211, 12th World AIDS Conference, Geneva, Switzerland, June 23-July 3, 1998.

12

CHILDREN WITH
HEPATITIS B
A Growing Problem

Two years ago, I went to Vietnam to adopt a five-month-old baby. Nobody was more surprised than I was when Jon's blood test results came back. The nurse called and said he tested positive for hepatitis B.

I looked up hepatitis B in the baby book, and it said, "Hepatitis B is an often fatal liver disease in children." I was devastated. I started to cry. It was awful.

I had been worried about attachment disorder because Jon was having trouble bonding, but my first thought was, "He's mine." It was an instantaneous conversion. We just bonded.

Karen

WHEN CHILDREN HAVE a serious infection like hepatitis B, it affects the whole family. Mothers feel a profound sense of guilt if they passed the virus to their babies. Parents who adopt children from countries with high rates of hepatitis B may find themselves dealing with a potentially serious infectious illness.

When I adopted my baby and then found out he had hepatitis B, I stayed up most of the night looking for information on the Internet.

There's not a wealth of specific information for kids. Our pediatrician didn't know much either.

But the public health department called right away. And a week later they sent me a letter wanting to know who my son's sexual partners were. He's five months old.

Joy

Researchers are just beginning to study treatment in children, so current information is often vague and indefinite. And that adds to a parent's anxiety. As a parent, you feel concerned about your family—and you're concerned about yourself, too, if you're ill with hepatitis B.

A diagnosis of hepatitis B is extremely stressful for parents. According to Marjanne Claassen, R.N., M.S., C.N.S., Clinical Nurse Specialist and Pediatric Liver Center Coordinator in the Section of Pediatric Gastroenterology, Hepatology, and Nutrition at Denver's Children's Hospital, "An adoptive parent may have been told the child is free of hepatitis B, then gets lab results that show the child does have the virus. Then there is the mother who transmitted the infection to her baby. Three to five percent of babies who get hepatitis B vaccine and HBIG (hepatitis B immune globulin) at birth still become positive, and the mothers have to deal with complex emotional issues, guilt issues."

How do infants get hepatitis B? Babies become infected usually in one of two ways: (1) when the mother passes the infection to her baby at birth (commonly referred to as vertical transmission), and (2) through contact with other infected siblings, household contacts, or playmates (commonly referred to as horizontal transmission).

In some parts of the world (Southeast Asia, China, Phillipines, sub-Saharan Africa) up to 10 to 30 percent of infants are infected. Be sure that tests for hepatitis B have been performed when considering adoption of a child from a region of the world where hepatitis B is widespread, but know that the results may not be reliable. Your child should be retested upon arrival in the United States. Family members and caretakers should be immunized with the hepatitis B vaccine.

Resource: To find out where to go for vaccinations, call the CDC National Immunization Hotline (800-232-2522) or your local or state health department. Vaccines are usually free for children when families can't afford them. For Spanish language inquiries, call 800-232-0233.

After birth, young children may become infected with hepatitis B through exposure and close personal contact with infected siblings, household contacts, or playmates. It is hoped that the current practice of universal vaccination against hepatitis B will eliminate this mode of transmission.

Exposure to blood or blood products can be another way to acquire hepatitis B infection. However, current tests used to screen blood donors are highly sensitive and specific and have nearly completely eliminated transfusion as a mode of transmission of hepatitis B in the United States. Prior to sensitive testing in 1975, transfusion of blood or blood products was considered a common risk for becoming infected with hepatitis B.

Adolescents may acquire hepatitis B through exposure to infected blood, sexual transmission, intravenous drug use, tattoos, skin piercing, and all the other ways adults become infected (see Chapter 3). This age group has its own problems with care and management of hepatitis B. However, issues regarding diagnosis, medical treatment, progression of liver disease, and transplantation are probably similar to the adult population, and I refer you to those topics in previous chapters.

Note: Discussions and recommendations in this chapter are meant as guidelines. Please consult your pediatrician, or your pediatric hepatologist or gastroenterologist regarding specific issues in treatment and management.

Here are the topics we'll cover:

- Overview
- Does Your Child Have Hepatitis B?
     Hepatitis B Surface Antigen (HBsAg) Testing
     Antibody Testing
     HBV DNA and e antigen (eAg) Testing
     Can Infection Be Prevented?
- Should Women with Hepatitis B Avoid Pregnancy or Breastfeeding?
- Can Your Child Participate in Regular Activities?
     Disclosure: To Tell Or Not To Tell?
     Chronic Disease and Your Family
     Resources for Parents
          Online Support Groups
          Resource for Healthy Eating
     Resources for Children
          On Hepatitis

Overview

The United States has a low prevalence of hepatitis B (approximately 0.5 percent of the population). Thirty percent of new infections are acquired at or around the time of birth (vertical transmission) or during early childhood (horizontal transmission), and 70 percent are acquired in adolescence or adult life. Adolescent and adult cases are usually due to transmission via blood, blood products, use of needles (intravenous drug abuse), or sexual exposure.

"If a baby is born to a mother with hepatitis B who is e antigen positive and the baby receives no treatment, the baby's risk of developing chronic hepatitis B is 70 percent, according to the Centers for Disease Control and Prevention," says Dr. Michael R. Narkewicz, M.D., Section of Pediatric Gastroenterology, Hepatology and Nutrition, Hewit/Andrews Chair in Pediatric Liver Disease, and Medical Director of the Denver Children's Hospital Pediatric Liver Center. "If the baby gets HBIG but no vaccine, the risk of developing chronic hepatitis B drops to 50 percent. If the baby gets vaccine and HBIG, the risk of developing chronic hepatitis B is to 3 to 4 percent. If the baby receives just the vaccine, the risk is 8 percent. It's clear that the most important thing is that the baby receives the vaccine. This is particularly important for infants born in countries with a high rate of hepatitis B."

One caveat: The current policies of testing pregnant women for hepatitis B, coupled with the administration of hepatitis B vaccine plus HBIG to the newborns, have eliminated about 90 to 95 percent of cases of vertical transmission in the United States. However, the CDC estimates that there are at least 150,000 pregnancies each year in the U.S. in women who emigrated from regions of the world with a high prevalence of hepatitis B. The risk of vertical transmission of hepatitis B will rise as the number of immigrants from these regions of the world increases, especially if these populations lack access to health care, hepatitis B vaccine and HBIG.

"The risk of developing chronic hepatitis B depends on the age when you get infected," says Dr. Narkewicz. "The earlier you acquire the infection, the less likely you are to be clinically sick, but the more likely you are to go on to a chronic infection. For example, a baby infected with HBV at birth almost never has clinical symptoms, but 90 percent of babies infected at birth develop a chronic infection with hepatitis B. If you acquire the infection at one year of age, you have about a 50 percent chance of developing chronic hepatitis B. The risk of developing chronic hepatitis B following an acute hepatitis B infection continues to drop as you get older until you reach five years of age, when the risk is 5 to 10 percent, which is similar to that of adults."

I would like to emphasize one point about perinatal or vertical transmission. It is clear that a mother with hepatitis B may transmit the virus to her infant at the birth of the newborn. However, not all newborns will become infected. The risk of vertical transmission is directly related to the degree of viral replication of hepatitis B in the mother. It is greatest (approaching 85 percent) when the mother is positive for e antigen and HBV DNA but lower (approximately 15 percent) when the mother is negative for e antigen and HBV DNA. All of these newborns, however, should be treated with vaccine plus HBIG, regardless of the e antigen and HBV DNA status of the mother. (For more information on the hepatitis B vaccine and HBIG, see Chapter 8.)

Mothers with chronic hepatitis B who are co-infected with HIV typically have higher levels of circulating hepatitis B virus. Therefore, infants born of these mothers are at higher risk of becoming infected with hepatitis B. Although the effectiveness of treating these babies with vaccine plus HBIG is unknown, these babies should receive vaccine and HBIG. If the infant becomes co-infected with HIV and hepatitis B, the immune response to the vaccine may be impaired, limiting the vaccine's effectiveness in preventing hepatitis B infection at or around the time of birth.

"Although children account for only about five percent of acute hepatitis B infection in the United States," says Dr. Narkewicz, "they account for about 25 percent of patients chronically infected with hepatitis B. This is an argument for targeting children for hepatitis B vaccination."

Does Your Child Have Hepatitis B?

Most infants who become acutely infected with hepatitis B don't show any specific signs or symptoms of hepatitis. For this reason, we depend upon specific viral tests.

Hepatitis B Surface Antigen (HBsAg) Testing. This is the test most commonly used to document transfer of infection from mother to infant. A newborn with positive hepatitis B surface antigen is infected with hepatitis B.

Antibody Testing. Because antibodies may not indicate active infection, antibody testing is not used to document transmission of infection to the newborn. Mothers with chronic hepatitis B have circulating antibodies against core and e antigen. These hepatitis B antibodies (HBcAb and HBeAb) in the mother's blood cross the placental barrier and are detected in the baby's blood. This movement of the mother's antibodies to the baby is called passive transfer and does not mean that the virus itself has transferred to the baby. Passively acquired antibodies usually persist for six to twelve months and never beyond fifteen months.

HBV DNA and e Antigen (eAg) Testing. We assess viral replication and activity of infection by measuring HBV DNA and e antigen in infants who are positive for hepatitis B surface antigen. Positive e antigen and HBV DNA indicate ongoing infection and active viral replication.

Can Infection Be Prevented? As previously emphasized, infection can be prevented in over 90 percent of cases using the combination of hepatitis B vaccine plus HBIG administered to the newborn immediately after delivery. Vaccine doses are then repeated at one to two months and six months. Effective vaccination also eliminates the risk of subsequent transmission with exposure to hepatitis B.

Despite HBIG and vaccine, some newborns still become infected. These children should be closely monitored by their pediatrician and referred to a pediatric gastroenterologist or hepatologist who will follow their cases and determine if they are candidates for interferon or other antiviral therapies.

Should Women with Hepatitis B Avoid Pregnancy or Breastfeeding?

The decision to proceed with childbearing is personal and individual. Most experts in this field conclude that women with hepatitis B should not avoid pregnancy simply because they have hepatitis B, even though there is the potential risk of transmitting the virus to their infant.

I got pregnant with twins. The first words out of my obstetrician's mouth were, "You'll probably need to have an abortion because of the hepatitis B." I consulted an infectious disease specialist who said no, just have the babies vaccinated within 12 hours and give them HBIG.

Both children had neonatal jaundice. It scared me, but the jaundice wasn't due to hepatitis B and cleared right up. Then we had to make sure they got their additional shots at one month and six months. We had to wait six months to check their antibody levels. Thank God they were okay.

Della

The overall risk of transmission from a mother who is positive for hepatitis B surface antigen, e antigen negative, and DNA negative to her newborn is about 15 percent, and the risk for an e antigen positive and DNA positive mother is about 80 percent in the absence of treatment with vaccine plus HBIG. Treatment with vaccine plus HBIG is more than 90 percent effective. So, with treatment, the overall risk of a baby becoming infected with hepatitis B is about 3 to 5 percent.

The potential for transmission of hepatitis B through breastfeeding is virtually eliminated by successful treatment of the newborn with vaccine and HBIG. "The official recommendation from the American Academy of Pediatrics is that breastfeeding of the infant (who has been vaccinated) by a hepatitis B surface antigen positive mother poses no additional risk for acquisition of HBV infection by the infant," adds Dr. Narkewicz.

Can Your Child Participate in Regular Activities?

Hepatitis B is not spread by casual contact, and children with the virus may participate in all regular activities, including school, play, day care, child care, extracurricular activities, and sports. One exception would be the child infected with hepatitis B who also has active dermatitis or skin wounds and sores. Such a child should not participate in sports involving close physical contact, such as wrestling, until the condition heals.

Tell your child that he or she cannot give hepatitis B to friends, classmates, family, or other acquaintances by sneezing, coughing, holding, hugging, or kissing; by sharing food, water, eating utensils, or drinking glasses; or by any other casual contact. The Centers for Disease Control guidelines don't disqualify anyone from school unless they show aggressive behavior, such as biting or scratching.

The disease can be spread by blood exposure, so cuts or abrasions should be carefully cleaned and bandaged to avoid contact with other children. In addition, the child should be told to avoid putting his or her fingers in other children's mouths (in order to prevent possible biting), sharing toothbrushes and razor blades, and making other contact with open sores or wounds.

> *My eight-year-old son knows he has a liver disease, and he knows never to touch another person's blood. We tell him to keep his blood private, and we give him examples of what to do in case of emergencies both for himself and for others. We rehearse the reaction so if it happens, there's more chance that he'll know what to do.*
>
> *If a friend is hurt, he shouldn't try to mend or touch the bleeding cut. There are other ways to help. He should run and get help. On the flip side, if he is hurt, he can apply pressure to the cut, wrap clothes around it. He shouldn't let someone else touch his cut.*
>
> *Ann*

Parents will be pleased to know that in December 2000, the American Academy of Pediatrics (AAP) announced that athletes with HIV, HBV, or HCV should be allowed to participate in all sports and that doctors should maintain patient confidentiality. The AAP policy statement states that there is a "very low probability" that these infections would be transmitted among young athletes. The AAP recommends that athletic programs promote hepatitis B vaccination, use Occupational Safety and Health Administration (OSHA) Universal Precautions, and inform students and parents that there is a "very small but finite risk" of a blood-borne infection.

Resource: To read the entire policy statement, go to the AAP Website: www.aap.org/policy/re9821.html.

Disclosure: To Tell Or Not To Tell? As a parent, one of the major problems you face is disclosure. It's important to tell doctors and dentists about your child's condition, but do you tell the daycare facility, the school, caregivers, friends? Here are some nurses' and parents' opinions:

"There is a disparity between the ideal and the real situation," says Claassen. The approach in schools is to use standard precautions. The ideal is that every staff member will deal with every child's blood in the same protective way. The OSHA standards for Universal Precautions say that all blood is assumed to be contaminated. Therefore, the school worker must assume that there are germs in everybody's blood, and of course with any blood-borne illness most children have it well before anyone knows they have it.

"Protective Personal Equipment (PPE—disposable protective gloves) is usually all that's needed. Because of standard precautions, the family has no *legal* obligation to tell anyone a child's diagnosis. In addition, everyone in school should be protected by required hepatitis B immunization. Standard precautions and immunization should decrease parents' anxiety. That's the ideal.

"The reality is that the parent usually chooses to tell the school. I recommend that families notify the professional registered nurse in charge of their child's school. A registered nurse understands the issues of confidentiality and will be prepared to handle questions as they come up."

When I first got the news in January, I told the daycare provider. I was worried that she'd quit, but she was great. She went to get the vaccination—which relieved my anxiety. Plus her insurance covered the shot.

I have the philosophy that a teacher or coach probably has been vaccinated for hepatitis B. If a blood spill happened, I'd call and have a discussion about the vaccine.

I'm more worried about her church group. Game time can get kind of wild. I said I'd be there and have gloves—just in case. I'm not worried about the kids; kids are supposed to be vaccinated. If they aren't, it's the parents' choice. But I do worry about a Good Samaritan adult who might step in case of an accident.

My daughter Lia went to a small preschool. I told them that her little brother had hepatitis B because it was stressful for Lia. I wanted her teachers to know. They said they had a previous child with HBV and at that time they sent a letter home to all the parents without naming the child.

Well, we live in a small town. It's not hard to figure out who it could be. So I called the public health department, and they said we don't have to inform others because the school is supposed to use Universal Precautions.

I'm careful about who knows. I told friends, family, and my childcare provider and didn't have a problem. Everyone was—and is—supportive.

"Be knowledgeable yourself," says Nancy Butler-Simon, M.S., R.N., C.N.S., C.P.N.P., Advanced Practice Nurse at Denver Children's Hospital's Pediatric General Clinical Research Center. "Daycare providers should get vaccinated and have their antibody levels checked to make sure they are protected. As the child gets older, be right up front with the school nurse. Have a script. Educate people. The school nurse can help you do that. Panic is the most contagious thing on this planet; deal with it by teaching others. Nip anxiety in the bud with knowledge."

Aside from school, parents and children must also decide what friends to inform and how. Parents must find the balance between secrecy and privacy. If people don't know much about hepatitis B, they might become alarmed.

We told six families. One family pretty much instantly stopped seeing us. They were the ones who picked us up at the airport at 4 a.m. the day we returned from Poland with our adopted child, and they had tears in their eyes. But from the day I told them, the door closed—no words, no discussion. Our kids don't play together. We're not invited to dinner.

The other five families have been terrific. One family watched all four of our kids so we could vacation. They told us their kids were vaccinated, and they take Universal Precautions.

Mona

It's important to communicate that hepatitis B is not transmitted casually but through blood, sex, contaminated needles, and from a mother with HBV to her newborn at birth. Household contacts are at risk primarily if they provide care to the infected individual or share sharps or hygienic utensils (razor blades, scissors, nail clippers, toothbrushes, etc). Tell people that a safe hepatitis B vaccine exists.

As children approach adolescence, parents should discuss decisions about future behaviors. Ideally, the topics of body piercing, tattooing, illegal drugs, and safe sex will be introduced in the context of family values when children are young. Pre-adolescence is an opportunity to make youngsters aware that you can not only give diseases like hepatitis B and AIDS, you can also get these illnesses from these exposures.

Hepatitis B is a sexually transmitted disease. Sexual organs are vascular. They have many blood vessels so that body fluids from these organs (vaginal secretions and semen) contain virus due to contamination with blood or serum. Less vascular tissues like the secreting glands of the eyes (tears) and salivary glands of the mouth (saliva) are less likely to have blood or serum contamination. "That's why we are more concerned about transmission through semen, more than tears," says Claassen, "vaginal secretions, more than saliva."

According to Butler-Simon, it helps to rehearse possible scenarios. "It's like teasing. If you ask your son if he's being teased, he has to admit that he's one-down. But if you ask if there is a bully on the playground, you open the possibility of a helpful discussion. It's in how you ask. Don't say, 'Are you having sex with Jane?' Instead ask, 'Is there anyone in your class who is already having sex?' Then your child can say, 'Yes, I know someone,' and you can ask, 'What do you think?' You are giving him the okay, the message that you are a safe listener. This can lead into what you need to do to protect yourself and others from pregnancy, AIDS, and hepatitis B."

In summary, says Claassen, "Think carefully before you share your child's diagnosis. The fear of hepatitis B is subsiding, but it's not gone. Balance responsibility with caution and with making your child's life as normal as possible. You don't want a big red 'H' on your child's head."

> *Resource:* Many organizations offer information to parents. Some also provide sample letters that can be given to schools. Contact the American Liver Foundation, Hepatitis B Coalition, Hepatitis B Foundation, and Parents of Kids with Infectious Diseases (see the Resources section at the end of this book).

Chronic Disease and Your Family. Hepatitis B affects everyone in the family—in positive as well as negative ways (see Chapter 5). Whom do you tell and when do you tell them? Brothers and sisters worry about the sick sibling but may be jealous over the extra attention paid to the child with hepatitis B.

Tammy was five when this whole thing started with her little brother. The first couple of months after the diagnosis, I was trying to figure out what to do, and I was stressed, worried.

Tammy is intelligent and energetic. She doesn't like not getting her full share of my attention. I was in crisis, and she wasn't giving me a break. I yelled a lot and took a lot out on her. Once I settled down, got the information, and started talking to her, things got better.

I told her that Ricky has some germs in his blood, and we're giving him shots to get rid of the germs. I also told her to be careful if Ricky was bleeding.

After that, Tammy somehow knew she had to take a back seat. She was very helpful with the shots and nice to her brother after the shot was over. Now that the crisis is past, she is saying, "You love Ricky more," and so on. She's doing all that normal sibling rivalry thing now!

Shelly

Another big issue is body image. Children don't like to feel different. Sometimes, even if they have no symptoms of hepatitis B, they may think they look different. Talk to your children. Let them tell you their fears. Reassure them. Above all, your child needs to know that hepatitis B is a medical condition, not a reason to feel ashamed.

Chronic disease is a strain, emotionally and financially. Your pediatrician and local children's hospital have resources to help you: social workers, specialists in financial matters, nurses and doctors who've dealt with the same problems you're facing. Talking to others can help you keep your perspective.

At the liver clinic I saw little kids with shunts. Those poor kids. Then my friend's child died of cancer at age 10. It put it in perspective for me. My son is not facing imminent death. Hepatitis B is not great, but it's not the worst thing that can happen to a kid.

Another friend had a child who was born blind. She gave me some good advice. "Don't be so worried about the future that you miss out on what you've got now," she said, because she feels she lost the first two years of her daughter's life. So I'm enjoying my son. He's healthy and active.

We had five boys, and we wanted a girl. The only way to be sure we'd have a girl was to adopt. It took us two years, and we went through three social workers.

Finally, the agency said we have a little girl in Romania "just to die for." They sent a video. She stole our hearts.

Then we got her hepatitis B medical records, but she was in our hearts. She was our girl.

Resources for Parents: Organizations listed in Resources at the back of this book provide avenues to support groups, online chat groups, videotapes, research archives, and educational packets; they also offer helpful material specifically for parents and children, including parents of adopted children from abroad. In addition, about a dozen children's hospitals now have international adoption clinics that offer counseling on medical, developmental, and attachment issues. Your local children's hospital library also is a good source of information, or you can go online to Hepatitis B Research Archives and use the search engine to find articles on children: http://dispatch.mail-list.com/archives/hbv_research/

Call the CDC's Immunization Hotline or your local or state health department to find out where you can go for vaccinations, which are usually free for children when families can't afford them: 800-232-2522; for Spanish language inquiries, call 800-232-0233.

Online Support Groups.
The Hepatitis B Foundation lists the following hepatitis B online support groups for parents and patients in its newsletter, *B-Informed:*
Hepatitis B Information and Support List:
   http://www.geocities.com/Heartland/Estates/9350/hblist.html
   To subscribe, send a blank email to: hepatitis-b-on@mail-list.com
HBV Adoption Support List: (for all parents of children with HBV):
   http://www.onelist.com/community.hbv-adoption
   To subscribe, go to www.onelist.com/subscribe/hbv-adoption
PKIDs Support List for parents (kids are encouraged to participate)
   and research archives: http://www.pkids.org
Resource for Healthy Eating. A low-fat, balanced, healthy diet is appropriate for people with liver disease (see Chapter 5). Note: Parents of children with cirrhosis should consult their doctors about dietary restrictions.

For a free copy of the colorful *Tips for Using the Food Guide Pyramid for Young Children 2 to 6 Years Old* (with recipes), contact The U.S. Department of Agriculture, Center for Nutrition Policy and Promotion: 202-606-8000. Website: www.usda.gov/cnpp

Resources for Children:

On Hepatitis:

Aronson, Virginia. *Everything You Need to Know About Hepatitis.* New York: Rosen Publishing Group, 2000 (middle school, high school).

Silverstein, Alvin, Virginia, & Robert. *Hepatitis.* Springfield: Enslow Publishers, 1994 (middle school, high school).

The American Digestive Health Foundation offers a free interactive computer game on CD-ROM, "Hepachallenge," which deals with prevention of hepatitis. (adolescents). To order, call 1-800-668-5237. Other interactive games and quizzes with an animated superhero help educate young teens about hepatitis B and the liver at www.HepBinfo.com

On General Issues of Chronic Illness:

Heegard, Marge. *When Someone Has a Very Serious Illness.* Mpls.: Woodland Press, 1991 (workbook for preschool and elementary school children).

Huegel, Kelly. *Young People and Chronic Illness (True Stories, Help, and Hope).* Mpls.: Free Spirit, 1998 (middle school, high school).

LeVert, Suzanne. *Face to Face with Chronic Illness.* New York: Messner/Simon & Schuster, 1993 (high school).

Moe, Barbara. *Coping with Chronic Illness.* New York: Rosen Publishing Group, 1992 (middle school, high school).

Band-aids and Blackboards. A colorful Website about growing up with medical problems with areas for kids, teens, and adults: http://funrsc.fairfield.edu/~ifleitas/contents.html

On Children Facing Liver Transplants:

Murphy-Melas, Elizabeth. *Pennies, Nickels & Dimes.* Santa Fe: Health Press, 1999.

Ribal, Lizzy. *Lizzy Gets a New Liver/Lizzy Tiene un Higado Nuevo.* Louisville: Bridge Resources, 1997.

Shadow Buddies. A Website that offers condition-specific dolls for your child, including one for liver transplant patients (complete with hospital gown, "Y" incision, and Hickman catheter), with a link to Shadow Buddies Foundation: www.shadowbuddies.com

The Course of the Infection in Children

The natural history or course of hepatitis B in children who acquire the disease vertically from the mother at the time of delivery is relatively well understood. A minority (less than 10 percent) develop clinical symptoms at the time of acute infection. About 90 percent of infections that are vertically-acquired result in chronic infection. In contrast, horizontally-acquired infection in children over age five, adolescents, and adults is more likely to cause jaundice or flu-like symptoms during acute infection, and less than 10 percent develop chronic infection. Horizontally-acquired infection between ages one to five carries intermediate risk of symptomatic acute disease and chronic infection.

Children with vertically-acquired infection are characterized by relatively high levels of circulating virus, positive e antigen, and positive HBV DNA, but they typically have normal ALT levels. A liver biopsy is not indicated in this setting. If performed, a liver biopsy usually would reveal little or no liver injury, but stains of the tissue would be markedly positive for hepatitis B. This situation is best described as immunologic tolerance; the patient lives with the virus, does not mount an immune reaction, and the liver is spared from injury. However, hepatitis B can integrate into the DNA of the patient and still cause genetic damage that, over years, can lead to liver cancer.

Studies of long-term outcome after infection in Chinese children (who generally acquire HBV vertically) indicate that about 30 percent of patients spontaneously seroconvert from e antigen to e antibody by 20 years of age. This change to the chronic carrier state is often heralded by a rise in ALT and is associated with the disappearance of HBV DNA from serum and a normalization of ALT. In contrast, children who acquired their chronic hepatitis B through horizontal transmission are more likely to have an immune response to the virus, and many have abnormal ALT levels. Biopsies show mild to moderate inflammation and relatively less staining of hepatitis B in liver cells.

Italian children, who represent a population with a greater proportion of horizontally acquired cases, have a different course. In long-term follow-up, as many as 70 percent seroconvert from e antigen to e antibody by 20 years of age. Reversion from e antibody to e antigen is rare, and sustained remission of disease activity is the rule. The differences in natural history of these two populations, Chinese and Italian, are thought to be related to differences in time of acquisition of infection, modes of transmission, viral factors, and host factors.

The vast majority of children with chronic hepatitis B have mild disease and few or no symptoms. Liver enzymes are typically normal or only slightly elevated. Liver biopsies usually demonstrate only mild degrees of inflammation or fibrosis. Progression of chronic hepatitis B to cirrhosis or development of liver cancer before age 18 is rare but does occur. Nonetheless, the chronically-infected child is at an increased risk for chronic active hepatitis, progression to cirrhosis, and the development of liver cancer and must be monitored.

The natural history or course of chronic hepatitis B in children and adolescents who acquire infection horizontally between ages 5 to 17, approximates the course in adults (see Chapters 1, 2, and 8).

Note: All patients with underlying liver disease, including hepatitis B, should get the hepatitis A vaccine. It is given in a two-part series starting at age 24 months. Consult your pediatrician, pediatric hepatologist or gastroenterologist.

Blood Draws and Biopsies

Practical Suggestions. When a child has hepatitis B, parents frequently have to prepare their child for painful procedures, such as blood draws and biopsies. According to Butler-Simon, emotional pain and physical pain are equally challenging and often inseparable. Doctors and nurses often underestimate pain. Parents know their children best and should speak up for them. Here are some of her practical suggestions:

- Use EMLA® Cream to numb the area before a blood draw. Left on the skin for an hour, it will numb the area up to a half-inch deep.
- Give Tylenol® beforehand (size and age-recommended dosage).
- Prepare the child beforehand, using language and concepts that are developmentally appropriate. Explain the procedure directly, honestly, simply.
- Bring something distracting with you—anything your child likes to hold, listen to, or watch.
- Teach your child to help themselves (Take an imaginary journey? Put on a "magic sock?").
- Offer choices. Which arm? Sit up or lie down?
- Use a "hug hold" to provide emotional support for a blood draw. Hold the child on your lap. You hug the child, and the child hugs you. Let the health care staff do the rest.

- For a biopsy, stronger medication is used to keep the child still and prevent pain. Stay close by and provide familiar comfort items to help the child relax.[1]

Encourage children to drink plenty of fluids before a blood draw. This is a simple but effective way to make it easier for the medical technician or nurse to find the veins.

Monitoring Children with Hepatitis B

According to Dr. Narkewicz, there are no standard recommendations. "Here at the Denver Children's Hospital Pediatric Liver Center, our recommendation is that the child should have liver blood tests performed once or twice a year (more frequently if the liver blood tests are abnormal), alpha-fetoprotein (tumor marker) every six months, and an ultrasound at a minimum of every two years or if the alpha-fetoprotein is rising. We follow the child's e antigen and antibody status every one to two years.

"Indications for treatment of HBV in children are abnormal liver blood tests, e antigen positive, and HBV DNA positive—persisting for greater than six months, and an abnormal liver biopsy consistent with hepatitis B."

Liver Biopsy. "I think liver biopsy is mandatory before deciding on a course of treatment," says Dr. Narkewicz, "because it tells us how much scarring has occurred in the liver and makes sure that the abnormal blood tests are the result of hepatitis B and not some other unsuspected liver disease.

"We do all our liver biopsies using the needle biopsy technique under sedation or anesthesia to make it more comfortable for the child, less anxiety-provoking, and to minimize risks. It is either a day procedure or a short overnight procedure. The major risk is bleeding so we always assess children's blood clotting level before a liver biopsy. The risk of significant bleeding in pediatric liver biopsies is about 1 to 3 percent."

Treatment

Jack's liver biopsy showed mild scarring and inflammation. In my mind, his liver was taking a hit. He was barely one year old, and his liver was already damaged.

When the pediatric hepatologist and I talked about treatment options, we decided to wait six months until Jack was older and bigger. The literature says to start at two years of age, but my doctor believes in treating early and aggressively.

I also wanted to contact the adoption agency for more information. If my son got infected in utero, the chances of his clearing the virus were not good. If he got it in the orphanage, the chances improved.

I found out via the grapevine that three babies and the caretaker in his room tested positive. They had told me Jack tested negative at three months and right before I got him. Either they falsified the tests or the orphanage used the same needle on other kids when they drew blood.

Conditions were primitive. They didn't have electricity or running water. They didn't sterilize needles. Vietnam is a poor country.

Susanne

Most children will never require treatment for hepatitis B. For those who do, the only FDA-approved treatment for chronic hepatitis B in children is interferon alfa-2b (INTRON® A, Schering-Plough). Lamivudine, which is FDA-approved for use in adults, is currently under investigation in a multicenter trial of children. Other treatments, such as adefovir dipovoxil, entecavir, and vaccine therapy are not yet in clinical trials in children at the time of this writing.

Indications for Interferon. Criteria for interferon therapy in children include a persistently abnormal ALT, positive e antigen, positive HBV DNA, and chronic hepatitis on liver biopsy.

"In the three largest clinical trials," says Dr. Narkewicz, "24 to 58 percent of children treated with interferon in dosages of 3 to 10 MU/m2 [Mega Units per meter squared (meter refers to the body surface area of the child)] three times a week for four to six months had sustained viral remission (normal ALT, e antigen negative, and negative HBV DNA) for six months or more post-treatment. Experience with children from Southeast Asia suggests that if they meet similar entry criteria for treatment, their response to interferon will be similar."

Sustained responders remain negative for e antigen and HBV DNA, normalize ALT, improve liver histology, and have a benign clinical course. Some of these patients will clear hepatitis B from their liver and lose hepatitis B surface antigen from their blood in long-term follow-up. Some will develop hepatitis B surface antibody. Relapse of hepatitis B is rare after interferon-induced seroconversion from e antigen to e antibody. Liver disease in sustained responders ceases to progress. However, these children should continue to be monitored for liver cancer for their lifetimes.

In general, interferon therapy is well tolerated in children. Common side effects of interferon therapy are flu-like symptoms, hair loss (alopecia), malaise, fatigue, and low white blood cell counts. Thyroid disease, usually hypothyroidism, can be precipitated by therapy, and rare autoimmune reactions have been described. Neuropsychiatric symptoms (including depression and poor concentrating ability) occur but appear to be less frequent than in adults. Young children may experience growth retardation on therapy, but catch-up growth is the rule once treatment is discontinued.

Dana has always been low energy. Not any more. I was concerned because I had to sign her up for basketball before I knew she would start treatment. The games are Tuesday nights. The shot is Monday so every game is timed for the end of her "good" time when she is over the side effects.

I explained to her coach that Dana is taking some really nasty medicine, and if she seemed tired to let her rest for a while. So far, that hasn't happened.

The hardest part was seeing Mom as the villain giving the shot. For me it was seeing her sick. No one wants to see your little girl sick. She would complain and cry, "My head hurts so bad I can't even look."

Danny started a six-month course of interferon. It didn't really affect him. He never missed a day of playing or school. You would never have known he was on interferon.

My folks came out to help the first week Tom got interferon. It was hard for the first two weeks, actually. He was up at night and had flu symptoms: fever, achiness. Then it didn't seem to bother him after that.

During interferon treatment, a variety of responses can be seen," says Claassen. "Sometimes liver enzyme tests show an elevation, which may actually be good. Interferon boosts the immune system to fight the virus so the AST and ALT may go up. It's frustrating and confusing for parents looking for a clear answer. Each child will take a unique path. I always tell parents that we cannot see that path ahead of time."

Interferon monotherapy (interferon alone) in the selected pediatric population is approximately as effective as the same treatment in adults. Unfortunately, 42 to 75 percent fail treatment and remain chronically infected. There is data that suggests that early treatment of chronic hepatitis B (before three years of age) is associated with a much higher response rate—50 to 80 percent. Children should be referred to and evaluated by a pediatric gastroenterologist or hepatologist with experience in managing interferon therapy in this unique population.

Giving Injections. If a family chooses interferon therapy, it raises complex emotional issues. The parent must administer an injection and then deal with interferon's side effects. No parent likes to poke a child with needles. Often, the mother has gone through treatment herself and knows what side effects her child is facing.

"I do the first dose in the clinic," says Claassen, "and we watch the child for a couple of hours. I have the parents inject me with a saline solution so they get over the fear of entering someone's body with a needle. It's a sacred barrier."

Butler-Simon recommends that the parent allow the nurse to give them a saline injection so they can see how small the needle is and how much easier a subcutaneous (under the skin) injection is than an intramuscular one. "Am I inflicting pain? No. And the parent can see and feel that I'm not. That's what parents freak out about—hurting the child."

"Many parents have given a shot before—to themselves if they have hepatitis B or to a pet," says Claassen. "But still, even with experience, giving a shot to one's own child is different. We go through the steps to help them gain confidence, and they give the first shot here."

Tools that help parents, such as EMLA® Cream or ice to numb the skin are like "training wheels," until the parent gains confidence. But it's a trade-off. EMLA cream must stay on the skin for an hour, and during that hour anticipation and dread increase.

"First and foremost," says Butler-Simon, "is setting the attitude of the parent. Kids will respond to the parent's attitude, which should be 'no big deal, and if it is, we'll work through it,' rather than 'I'm so sorry, dear, but we have to do it.'"

My daughter is ten. At that age, a sense of choice and control is important. I let her decide what time she wanted to take the shots. Each time, I get everything ready so she has less than one minute to worry. I call her from my bedroom, and she knows. We always do the shot in the same place. We never do it in her bedroom because her bedroom has to be a safe place.

Lisa

Many parents want guidance on the mechanics of administering the injection. "For really young children, infants to age three or four, it's best to give the shot in the butt," says Butler-Simon. "You can lay them in your lap with your leg over their legs, hanging them over your other leg or place them on their belly on a couch. Distraction helps. Give them a doll that they can give a 'shot' to at the same time to help them feel that they have some control. Praise and stickers are helpful, but then move on. Don't drag the ritual out to the nth degree because you have to do it so frequently.

"At ages four to five, children may be able to be more cooperative. To elicit a sense of control, you can encourage them to do the alcohol swab, for example. For young school-age children, a 'hug-hold' is a good option. You hold the child on your lap. The child hugs you, you hug the child, and another adult gives the shot."

"Sometimes," says Claassen, "you have to come up with a good hold and get it over with. We've never had anyone fail therapy because it involves shots!"

I had to perfect the single parent shot technique for my two-year-old. I got the shot ready. Then I flipped Jon on my lap so his butt was facing me. I put my elbow or forearm on his back and my right forearm below his buttocks. Or I'd put his two legs between mine. This actually worked better because it left me with one hand free. Then I'd twist my hand around and give the shot.

Meanwhile, his big sister kept him busy with M & Ms® on the front!

Mollie

Nonresponders. Treatment options for children who have failed to respond to interferon are limited. Some researchers have suggested that retreatment with higher doses of interferon for longer durations (up to one year) may be effective in 10 to 30 percent of children who have failed standard regimens. The safety and efficacy of this approach is unknown. In addition, even if retreated, the great majority of nonresponders will fail to clear the virus with this regimen. Also, side effects (particularly a low white count, low platelet count, and growth retardation) limit the usefulness of this approach. In general, nonresponders must await the results of clinical trials of new therapeutic regimens.

> *Jan finished interferon a year ago. She still has the e antigen; she didn't seroconvert. But there's still a slight possibility it may happen yet. Meanwhile, the doctor says the interferon helped her liver.*
>
> *I was really disappointed. I feel, though, that I've done all I could do. When something's wrong, I want to fix it. It's counter-intuitive for me to sit around. At our next visit with the hepatologist, I'm hoping it's time to start the next drug.*
>
> *Ellen*

Lamivudine. Lamivudine is FDA-approved for treatment of chronic hepatitis B in adults (see Chapter 8) but not in children. It is highly effective in suppressing the replication of hepatitis B, and nearly 100 percent of patients treated with lamivudine clear HBV DNA from serum. Seroconversion from e antigen to e antibody occurs in 15 to 20 percent of cases.

The advantages of lamivudine over interferon alfa are that it's taken orally and doesn't seem to have significant side effects. The limitations of lamivudine are a rebound of hepatitis after treatment is discontinued, recurrence of hepatitis B in most cases, and development of mutations (see Chapter 8, YMDD mutations) in the hepatitis B viral genome that render the virus resistant to lamivudine.

Approximately 30 percent of patients who are treated with lamivudine for one year will develop YMDD mutations. These mutations are sensitive to adefovir dipivoxil. Currently, there is an ongoing U.S. multicenter trial of lamivudine in the treatment of chronic hepatitis B in children. At the time of this writing, the results of the trial have not yet been published.

Future Therapy. A number of new drugs and treatment strategies are in development or clinical trials in adults (see Chapters 8 and 13). Modified interferon (pegylated interferon) is just now receiving approval by the FDA. This form of interferon is long acting, requires only one injection a week, and may be preferred over standard interferon, which is given three times a week. Promising treatments include adefovir dipivoxil, entecavir, and vaccine therapy. Some of these treatments will undoubtedly soon be available for use in adults. It is likely that many will find their way to the treatment of pediatric cases.

Other promising approaches include combinations of interferon with nucleoside analogues (lamivudine, ribavirin, others) and vaccines that stimulate the immune response despite the fact that these patients already harbor chronic infection. The future of treatment holds great hope for patients and families currently dealing with chronic hepatitis B.

> *Resource:* For news of clinical trials for hepatitis B in children, contact Parents of Kids with Infectious Diseases (PKIDs) at 360-695-0293. Website: www.pkids.org
>
> *Resource:* Other Websites that track clinical trials include www.centerwatch.com and the National Institutes of Health Website: www.cc.nih.gov.
>
> *Resource:* The American Liver Foundation created a national Pediatric Liver Research Agenda under the leadership of Ronald Sokol, M.D., Director of The Children's Hospital Pediatric Liver Center, Professor of Pediatrics at the University of Colorado Medical School. Website: www.liverfoundation.org/html/advores.htm

Post-Treatment Follow-Up. Responders to interferon should be monitored for complete resolution of markers of viral infection. Nearly all responders will remain negative for e antigen and HBV DNA. Some will clear hepatitis B surface antigen, and some will even develop hepatitis B surface antibodies.

Children who have cleared e antigen but not surface antigen should still be monitored for development of liver cancer with alpha-fetoprotein every six months and serial ultrasonography. It is likely that the risk of cancer is reduced in these patients. However, the risk of cancer, especially in cirrhotics, is still high and screening is recommended. Nonresponders to therapy should be monitored for disease progression (see Monitoring Children with Hepatitis B).

Cirrhotic patients need to be watched for early signs of liver decompensation (see Chapter 4). These patients are at greatest risk for development of liver cancer (the estimated risk is approximately two percent per year) because they have both cirrhosis and active viral replication. Evidence of decompensation or development of isolated hepatoma (liver cancer) are indications for referral for liver transplantation.

Despite these concerns and the need for monitoring, most children with chronic hepatitis B have a relatively benign course with few symptoms and slow progression of liver disease. Time is on their side as treatment options expand, and the likelihood of cure with medical therapy becomes increasingly possible.

A child is one who stands halfway between an adult and a TV set.

Anonymous

Reference
[1] Liver Center and Liver Transplantation Program of The Children's Hospital (Denver). "Preparing Children for Painful Procedures," *Connections*, Fall/Winter 2000, Vol.13, No. 4:4–5.

1 3

RESEARCH TRENDS
Hope for the Future

People with hepatitis live life on a roller coaster. Some days are good, and you can almost forget that you're battling a chronic infection. Other days pass in a fog of fatigue and despair.

Each small step, each advance in research strengthens hope. The future looks promising, but we know that hepatitis B doesn't get much press, and that we need more research dollars.

Here's where we can do something. Each of us can talk about hepatitis B and increase awareness. Each of us can contribute time and money to finding the cure.

It's scary to know that a virus is circulating in your body, and that you can't get rid of it. Present therapies work for some people—but all of us feel that there's got to be something better coming down the pike. And we wait and hope.

Hedy

AS A HEPATOLOGIST counseling patients with hepatitis B, I find it frustrating not to have more tools to treat my patients. Even with the best antiviral regimen, the majority of hepatitis B patients fail to respond. Antiviral research is in its pioneering stage. I look forward to the next few years, and I expect to see exciting new advances.

Hepatitis B research falls into two broad and somewhat overlapping categories: clinical research and basic research. Clinical research primarily determines whether new drug therapies are effective in treating hepatitis B. Basic research encompasses a wide variety of studies of hepatitis B, including but not limited to molecular biology, cell biology, transplantation, pathophysiology, and pharmacology.

In this final chapter, we'll cover the following topics:

- Clinical Research: Testing New Drugs
    - *Phases of Clinical Trials*
    - *Should You Sign Up for a Study?*
- Current Clinical Research for Treatment of Hepatitis B
    - *Interferon-alfa*
    - *Long-Acting Interferons: Pegylation (PEG)*
    - *Thymosin-alpha1*
- Potential New Therapies
    - *Standard Vaccines*
    - *Vaccines for Treatment of Chronic Hepatitis B*
    - *Nucleoside/nucleotide analogues*
        - Adefovir
        - Entecavir
        - Emtricitabine
        - Others
    - *Ribozymes*
- Basic Research
    - *Molecular Virology*
    - *Cell Biology*
    - *Liver Cell Transplantation*
    - *Stem Cells*
    - *Pathophysiology*
    - *Pharmacology*
    - *The Bioartificial Liver*
- Research Funding

Clinical Research: Testing New Drugs

In the United States, pharmaceutical companies, the National Institutes of Health, and university medical centers test promising new drugs and submit their results to the Food and Drug Administration (FDA). It is the responsibility of the FDA to critically examine the results of the studies and determine whether the new treatment is safe and effective through a careful system of checks and balances. State review boards also monitor studies and adverse reactions to medications. Drugs approved by the FDA become available to practicing physicians to use in the treatment of hepatitis B.

A well-defined process evaluates all new drugs. First, the drug's safety must be established through animal testing. These studies may also help to define the expected effectiveness and dose ranges of the drug when it is used later in humans. After a drug has undergone animal testing and has been approved by the FDA for clinical research with humans, the drug testing enters three phases.

Phases of Clinical Trials. Studies in Phase I (human toxicity) typically involve small numbers of patients or healthy individuals who are given single doses of the drug in varying amounts. Study subjects are monitored very closely (physical examinations and blood testing) to detect any adverse effect of the medication. Researchers examine the absorption of the drug, its distribution in the body, metabolism, and elimination. Sometimes the cumulative toxicity of multiple doses of drug are examined in Phase I studies.

Phase II (dose finding) studies evaluate the response of the disease to the drug in large numbers of study subjects. Researchers determine the effectiveness of several different doses of the drug administered over prolonged periods of time to find the "optimal dose" for use in humans. Patients are also carefully monitored for evidence of toxicity.

Phase III (pre-clinical testing) typically evaluates the treatment in hundreds to thousands of patients. Again, effectiveness and toxicity are carefully evaluated. Researchers often compare the drug under investigation to existing therapies and medications to obtain a measure of whether the new treatment represents an advance above current treatment strategies. These are the final studies done to obtain FDA approval and will determine how the drug is labeled. After this phase is completed, the results are submitted to the FDA for review. Although some drugs, such as those to treat cancer, AIDS, and ALS, are on a fast track for FDA approval, it may take approximately two years for other drugs to be approved. The FDA may approve the drug, reject it, or request more studies.

Ongoing clinical testing (post-marketing surveillance for problems that might arise) occurs after the FDA has approved the drug, usually for the first one to two years, and determines optimal ways to use the drug or new indications for using the drug.

Should You Sign Up for a Study? Obviously, before you enroll in a specific study, you should take time to review the patient informed consent document that you will have to sign. Be sure to ask how often you will see a doctor; doctor appointments vary at different study sites. You should also consider all the pros and cons of any study.

On the positive side:

1. You may get to try a new treatment that is not available through general clinical practice.
2. Typically, you would receive frequent examinations and careful follow-up.
3. Study coordinators will keep you informed about your status and progress.
4. Most studies are sponsored by pharmaceutical companies or by research grants, and typically your treatment is delivered without expense to you or your insurer. However, the degree of compensation can vary, and you (or your insurer) may be responsible for some of the bill. Some studies also give extra compensation to you for expenses related to travel to the study site or for the time you spent participating in the research.
5. Your participation is kept confidential. Representatives from the FDA or study sponsors, however, have the right to review your study record.
6. You reserve the right to stop treatment and withdraw from the study at any time.

On the negative side:

1. Testing programs are rigid. You must make the time commitment to follow the protocol exactly. For example, you'll have to show up at certain times for follow-up tests.
2. Clinical trials are usually blinded. That means that you won't know what you're getting in terms of dosage or placebo, for example. If you have been given a placebo, the pharmaceutical company may offer the active drug to you (free of charge) at the end of your participation in the trial if you completed the study.

3. Sponsors can stop the trials at any time.
4. You may experience undocumented side effects.
5. You must be prepared to reveal all aspects of your physical and emotional health.
6. You won't know the results of the whole study, or your individual results, until every participant has completed the protocol. It may take more than a year from your point of enrollment.

If you fail to meet criteria for entry into the controlled studies, it is still possible to be treated with investigational drugs through compassionate-use protocols. Typically, drugs available on a compassionate-use basis have been proven to be effective but have not yet received FDA approval. Physicians gain access to these drugs by contacting the pharmaceutical sponsor.

Resources: The National Institutes of Health manage a Website with descriptions of more than 4,000 federal and private clinical studies nationwide. You may browse by disease or sponsoring organization. Website: www.clinicaltrials.gov

Other Websites with clinical trial information are www.centerwatch.com and www.hivandhepatitis.com/hepb/trials_b.html.

Resources: Contact patient support organizations listed in the Resources section at the end of this book for information on drugs in development.

Resource: A 99-page online FDA publication, *From Test Tube to Patient: Improving Health Through Human Drugs,* describes the process of developing and testing new drugs. The report also provides information about specific drugs. Website:
www.fda.gov/cder/about/whatwedo/testtube.pdf

Resource: The Center for Drug Evaluation and Research's handbook goes through the steps for approval of a new drug and the FDA's monitoring of a drug once it has been approved. Website:
www.fda.gov/cder/handbook/startpag.htm

Current Clinical Research for Treatment of Hepatitis B

Optimum therapy for hepatitis B is under constant evaluation and reappraisal. One of the most exciting—and frustrating—parts of writing about clinical research is that by the time you read this chapter, researchers will be studying new treatments. At the time of this writing, however, the following drugs are under investigation

Interferon-alfa. As stated above, interferon-alfa is one of two treatments that are FDA-approved for use against chronic hepatitis B. Current research with standard interferon is focusing on novel methods of drug delivery, such as administration via nasal spray and unique dosing regimens. A recent example of the latter was the demonstration that prolonged interferon therapy for 12 years could ultimately eradicate chronic hepatitis Delta infection. Follow-up studies are needed to determine if this effect can be duplicated in larger numbers of patients.

Long-Acting Interferons: Pegylation (PEG). Pharmaceutical companies (Schering-Plough, Roche) have developed methods (pegylation) to modify the parent interferon molecule in order to retain antiviral activity yet deliver the active drug more slowly to the body—much like a time-release capsule. PEG is an acronym for polyethylene glycol, an inert substance that is eliminated via the urine and bile.

Advantages of pegylated interferons over standard interferons include maintaining a constant and prolonged antiviral effect and reducing the amount of injections needed. The long-acting forms need only weekly injections. In addition, the persistent and prolonged antiviral activity afforded by these agents may aid in overall clearance of the hepatitis B virus. Clinical trials of pegylated interferons as monotherapy and in combination with other agents (nucleoside analogues, thymosin-alpha1) are now in progress, and early results indicate an increased rate of viral clearance.

Thymosin-alpha1. Thymosin-alpha1, Zadaxin® (SciClone), used alone, has demonstrated partial success in eradicating hepatitis B. An initial trial compared the results of six months of thymosin-alpha1 given to seven patients to a placebo administered to five patients. Thymosin suppressed viral replication, improved ALT, and cleared hepatitis B as demonstrated by analysis of post-treatment liver biopsies. A larger study comparing 17 patients treated with thymosin to 16 receiving a placebo also suggested that thymosin could reduce the replication of HBV and normalize ALT.

Other studies of small numbers of subjects have given conflicting results. Nonetheless, thymosin has been approved for sale in 20 countries outside the U.S., principally for the treatment of chronic hepatitis B and chronic hepatitis C. Ongoing studies of thymosin in combination with other agents, including lamivudine and standard and pegylated interferons, are promising.

> *Resource*: Use the search engine on the Hepatitis B Research Archives to find articles pertaining to your research topic: http://dispatch.mail-list.com/archives/hbv_research.

Potential New Therapies

Standard Vaccines. Unlike the case of hepatitis C, effective vaccine exists that can protect the immunized patient against infection with hepatitis B. The challenge is to make this vaccine available to all regions of the world. Universal vaccination programs have been demonstrated to reduce disease, liver failure, and liver cancer related to hepatitis B. Cooperative programs through the World Health Organization have been instrumental in the initiation of universal vaccination in China and other regions with high prevalence of hepatitis B.

These vaccination programs, however, are extremely expensive and beyond the means of many countries. For this reason, researchers are developing novel approaches to the vaccination of large populations. One approach is to bioengineer plants, such as potatoes, that produce hepatitis B surface antigen and can enter the food chain naturally. Individuals ingesting these plants would theoretically mount an immune response to the hepatitis B surface antigen and become protected against infection with the virus. Although promising, this approach has yet to be tested in appropriately conducted clinical trials. It is hoped that continued progress will be assured by active participation of local governments with world health officials and organizations.

Vaccines for Treatment of Chronic Hepatitis B. Traditional vaccines are designed to protect a susceptible population from becoming infected with a virus. New vaccine strategies target patients who already have a chronic infection. The goal of vaccination of chronically infected patients is to stimulate specific immune responses that can lead to viral clearance.

The current vaccines under investigation target the body's lymphocytes to induce a special type of immunity ("cell-mediated"). One recent clinical trial examined the response to a vaccine (CY-1899) that incorporated parts of hepatitis B core protein designed to stimulate special lymphocytes (T cells) in 90 patients with chronic hepatitis B. This vaccine did initiate significant and specific T cell responses but there was no effect on ALT, viral serology, or liver disease. The induced T cell responses were much lower than those observed with spontaneous clearance of hepatitis B after acute natural infection. Current studies are examining the role of the combination of vaccine plus other antivirals in the treatment of chronic hepatitis B.

Another approach to the stimulation of active immunity against hepatitis B is the oral administration of viral proteins. In a recent pilot study, 15 patients with chronic hepatitis B were fed a mixture of pre-S1, pre-S2 and hepatitis B surface antigen three times a week for 20 weeks. Two-thirds normalized ALT, 60 percent had a marked reduction in HBV DNA levels, and 40 percent improved inflammation on liver biopsy. Patients relapsed once treatment was discontinued. Additional controlled trials will be necessary to prove whether these preliminary observations can be confirmed.

Additional therapies whose target is modulation of the immune response are under development or in early phases of clinical investigation. These therapies include monoclonal antibodies, interleukins, levamisole, cytotoxic lymphocyte epitope vaccination, and DNA vaccination.

Nucleoside/nucleotide analogues. It is likely that the first new agents to emerge from clinical trials for the treatment of chronic hepatitis B will be nucleoside analogues. However, it is not clear which of the emerging drugs will actually make it to the level of clinical practice. A case in point is lobucavir, a drug that had gone through extensive pre-clinical and clinical testing. Clinical development of lobucavir ceased due to demonstration of liver malignancies in rats (hepatomas) and gynecological malignancies in mice and rats (vaginal cancer).

Adefovir. Of the emerging nucleoside analogues, adefovir dipivoxil (the active molecule is adefovir, PMEA) is likely to be the first to gain approval by the FDA (see Chapter 8 for a full discussion of adefovir). Concerns regarding renal toxicity with higher doses (> 30 milligrams per day) have not been realized with the lower doses used to treat hepatitis B. However, use of adefovir will require dose adjustments for renal dysfunction and careful monitoring for untoward side effects.

Entecavir. Entecavir is an analogue of guanosine and potently suppresses the replication of a number of viruses including herpesviruses and hepatitis B. This drug is currently in phase I-II clinical trials. Preliminary reports indicate that entecavir is effective in both naive patients and in patients who have failed prior treatments, including a few patients with YMDD mutations (see Chapter 8). Other studies suggest that prior treatment with lamivudine may reduce the response to entecavir.

Emtricitabine (FTC). Emtricitabine is a fluorinated derivative of lamivudine with greater potency against hepatitis B. It is currently in phase I-II clinical trials. Because it is chemically similar to lamivudine, YMDD mutations which are resistant to lamivudine may also be resistant to emtricitabine. A preliminary report of a dose-ranging trial in 98 patients with chronic hepatitis B indicated that emtricitabine is highly effective in suppressing HBV DNA. The drug appeared to be safe and well-tolerated in doses effective in suppressing hepatitis B.

Others. A number of unique compounds are under development or in the early stages of clinical trials. Most are identified only by numbers or letters: BMS-200475, MCC-478, MIV 210, AT 61, DAPD, L-FMAU, and others. The role of these agents in the treatment of hepatitis B remains to be defined.

Ribozymes. This is an exciting new approach to the treatment of viral diseases and, potentially, even cancer. Ribozymes are synthesized in a special way to be complementary to specific regions of viral RNA or DNA. Once the ribozyme binds to the viral RNA or DNA, a process is activated to cut and inactivate the viral RNA. In cell culture experiments, ribozymes have demonstrated the ability to block viral replication and eradicate infection. Trials with these agents are just beginning, but initial trials of treatment of patients with chronic hepatitis B with HepBzyme™ (Ribozyme Pharmaceuticals, Inc.) will likely be initiated by the fall of 2001.

Basic Research

Molecular Virology. Researchers have made amazing advances in understanding the hepatitis B virus, in large part because of techniques available through the new scientific field of molecular biology. As a result, scientists have completely defined the genetic makeup of the hepatitis B virus. Despite these advances, however, we still lack basic information about the proteins produced by this virus and how these proteins interact with one another and with the host cell.

Current studies are evaluating the types and properties of the proteins produced by the hepatitis B genes. It is likely that these studies will unlock the mechanisms of viral protein assembly, viral formation, and secretion of the virus out of the liver cell into blood. Understanding these critical steps required to maintain the hepatitis B infection will allow scientists to develop medications or strategies to stop the virus from reproducing (replicating) and, ultimately, to eradicate the infection.

Additional studies are trying to define how the hepatitis B virus genes control and regulate the virus's production of proteins and allow the virus to copy its own genes to make new virus. Replication maintains the infection; without it, hepatitis B would disappear after a period of time. Scientists, therefore, are looking for keys to designing drugs that will stop viral replication.

Cell Biology. Despite what we do know about the hepatitis B genes and many of the proteins produced, little is known about the interaction between the hepatitis B virus and the liver cell. Future studies in this area should yield fruitful information for designing therapies, but right now many questions remain unanswered, including the following:

- What attracts hepatitis B to the liver and not to other tissues?
- How does hepatitis B bind to the surface of a liver cell and get into it?
- Once hepatitis B enters the liver cell, how does it survive?
- Why doesn't the liver cell simply swallow it up and digest it?
- What cellular systems in the liver cell are required to aid the replication of the virus?
- What are the key determinants of assembly of the viral proteins and genes to form an active infectious particle?
- What processes within the liver cell control the secretion of the viral particle out of the cell?

Liver Cell Transplantation. An emerging field that is extremely exciting for both research applications and potential therapies is the isolation, storage, and subsequent use of human liver cells. These techniques have only recently become available with the development of human liver cell banks.

It's possible to freeze and store (cryopreserve) human liver cells taken from several specimens of human livers recovered for use in organ transplantation but rejected due to fatty change or physical damage to the organ. After sterile preparation, cells may be stored in a specialized cryopreservation medium for later thawing and use. Thawed cells are subsequently infused into patients with acute fulminant liver failure. In some cases, this technique has been successful at reversing some of the complications of liver failure and temporarily sustaining life.

Despite these initial promising results, in no case has liver cell transplantation saved patients independent of liver transplantation. Nonetheless, human liver cells have many major potential useful research applications, especially for studying the molecular virology and cell biology of hepatitis B. It is anticipated that researchers will be able to define the entire life cycle of hepatitis B with appropriate experiments using these cells.

Stem Cells. Research into mechanisms and treatment of human disease is often compromised by inadequate supply or lack of access to appropriate human tissues. A goal of investigators has been to isolate cells within the mature human liver that can be stimulated to regenerate, allowing the production of large quantities of human liver cells that could be used to study the details of viral infection and to design effective, safe drugs. Searching the human liver for these cells seemed reasonable since the liver is known to regenerate after resection or liver transplantation.

At the time of this writing, stem cells had just been isolated from mature, adult human liver, patented (Incara Pharmaceutical Corporation), and clinical trials using these cells in patients with liver failure or certain genetic diseases were in development. Liver stem cells have also been isolated from immature, fetal livers but controversies regarding use of human fetal tissue are likely to limit the availability of these cells for research or clinical trials.

A promising new development has been the demonstration that certain cells can be isolated from bone marrow that have the ability to differentiate into liver and bile duct cells. If these initial observations can be confirmed and the function of the cells characterized, then human bone marrow from adult volunteers might serve as a source of human liver cells for both research and drug development.

Pathophysiology. One interesting feature of hepatitis B (and viral hepatitis in general) is that the hepatitis B infection probably is not sufficient to destroy or damage liver cells by itself. We don't fully understand the complex process of liver cell injury and the formation of fibrous tissue in the liver. Finally, repair mechanisms, such as liver regeneration, are poorly defined.

Many different laboratories are studying the effects of cofactors that may contribute to liver cell injury, fibrosis, regeneration, and progression to cirrhosis. These cofactors include processes such as excessive iron accumulation, oxidative stress, abnormal bile salts, and inflammatory mediators released by immune cells.

In the absence of effective therapies to eradicate hepatitis B, therapies that can modify basic mechanisms of cell injury and fibrosis may reduce the rate of progression to cirrhosis and the need for liver transplantation, slow the progression to liver failure, and reduce the rate of death from liver disease.

Pharmacology. As you can see, it's easy to understand that future treatment of hepatitis B could involve medications that target many different sites. I've briefly mentioned immune therapies and nucleoside/nucleotide analogues, which directly target the virus. Antiviral agents that interfere with the assembly or secretions of viral genes or proteins may soon be developed.

In the absence of effective antiviral agents, treatments could focus on the mechanisms of liver cell injury. Antioxidants might be used to reduce the risk of oxidative liver cell injury. Iron removal by phlebotomy (drawing blood) may reduce storage of iron within the liver, perhaps reducing liver cell injury. Specific drugs may be developed to inhibit liver fibrosis. Undoubtedly, numerous other points of attack will be defined as our knowledge expands in the fields of molecular virology, cell biology, and pathophysiology of chronic hepatitis B.

The Bioartificial Liver. Patients who suffer from chronic kidney failure have an option, short of transplantation, that prolongs life: dialysis. Unfortunately, patients with chronic liver disease do not have a comparable liver dialysis machine.

Recently, several laboratories have begun to examine the effectiveness of bioartificial livers. Like dialysis machines, the patient's blood is passed through a capillary system to filter and cleanse the blood. One sorbent-based system (HemoTherapies™) has recently been approved by the FDA for treatment of patients suffering from liver decompensation with encephalopathy and drug overdose. The machine is used to remove toxins and balance fluid, electrolytes, and glucose. Current randomized controlled trials will ultimately define the role and impact of this system in the management of patients with liver disease.

Other bioartificial livers have added liver cells (pig hepatocytes, transformed cells, human hepatoma cell lines) to the system. The liver cells may be necessary to make the system function more like a normal liver. Theoretically, these functioning liver cells should help detoxify the patient's blood. In addition, researchers have suggested that substances synthesized and secreted by the liver cells may gain entry back into the blood and further support the patient.

Conceptually, many of the aspects of the bioartificial liver machine are sound and make sense. On the other hand, many technical problems limit the success of these machines. In the first place, the liver cells survive for only a short period of time, and cartridges need to be replaced frequently. Second, the cost of performing the dialysis is excessive. Third, the capillary barrier between plasma and liver cells is great and does not duplicate the processes of exchange between normal blood and liver cells in the patient. Fourth, the safety of these devices is unproven. As of this writing, most bioartificial liver machines are still considered experimental.

Research Funding

It is my hope that we are entering a new era in the treatment of hepatitis B, where research may ultimately lead to discoveries of more effective treatments that benefit patients. Research into the basic mechanisms of hepatitis B replication and infection of the liver cell is absolutely essential, so that our understanding and treatment of this devastating disease may leap forward.

However, research funding for hepatitis B is still minimal. The hepatitis B vaccine, while highly effective in preventing infection, has made the public complacent to the ongoing dangers of HBV. According to the Hepatitis B Foundation, the reality is that each year new infections occur in more than 200,000 Americans, and 6,000 to 7,000 Americans become critically ill. "Funding for AIDS increased tenfold to two billion dollars in a decade. Funding for HBV, a disease which chronically infects 1.25 Americans and has been a major public health problem for more than 30 years, has not significantly increased and remains virtually frozen at twenty million plus."[1]

Clearly, hepatitis B patients, friends, and family members must focus attention on research. We must make it our top priority to confront, define, and eradicate this serious viral infection.

Where observation is concerned, chance favors only the prepared mind.

Louis Pasteur

Reference
[1] "Not To B Forgotten," *B Informed*, No. 27 Winter 2000:2.

Resources

Organizations

American Liver Foundation (ALF)
75 Maiden Lane, Suite 603
New York, NY 10038-4810
1-800-GO-LIVER
1-888-4-HEP-ABC
1-888-4-HEP-USA
Website: www.liverfoundation.org
Email: www.webmail@liverfoundation.org

Hepatitis B Foundation
700 East Butler Avenue
Doylestown, PA 18901-2697
215-489-4900
Website: www.hepb.org
Email: info@hepb.org

Hepatitis Education Project
4603 Aurora Avenue North
Seattle, WA 98103-6513
1-800-218-6932
206-732-0311
Email: hep@scn.org

Hepatitis Foundation International (HFI)
30 Sunrise Terrace
Cedar Grove, NJ 07009-1423
1-800-891-0707
Website: www.hepfi.org
Email: HFI@intac.com

Immunization Action Coalition
& the Hepatitis B Coalition
1573 Selby Avenue
Suite 234
St. Paul, MN 55104
651-647-9009
FAX: 651-647-9131
Website: www.immunize.org
Email: admin@immunize.org

Latino Organization for Liver Awareness (LOLA)
P.O. Box 842, Throggs Neck Station
Bronx, NY 10465
1-888-367-LOLA
718-892-8697
Website: www.lola-national.org
Email: mdlola@aol.com

Parents of Kids with Infectious Diseases (PKIDS)
P. O. Box 5666
Vancouver, WA 98668
1-877-55-PKIDS
360-695-0293
Website: www.pkids.org
Email: pkids@pkids.org

On-Line Hepatitis B Support Groups

Hepatitis B Information and Support List
http://www.geocities.com/Heartland/Estates/9350/hblist.html
To subscribe, send a blank email to: hepatitis-b-on@mail-list.com

HBV Adoption Support List
http://www.onelist.com/community.hbv-adoption
To subscribe, go to www.onelist.com/subscribe/hbv-adoption

(See Organizations for additional support groups.)

Government Agencies

Centers for Disease Control and Prevention (CDC)
1600 Clifton Road N.E.
Hepatitis Branch, Mailstop G37
Atlanta, GA 30333
CDC Hepatitis Hotline: 1-888-443-7232
CDC Public Inquiries: 1-800-311-3435
Website: www.cdc.gov/ncidod/diseases/hepatitis/
Email: dvd1hep@cdc.gov

Departments of Public Health
For information about hepatitis B in your state, call your State Department of Public Health, Epidemiology Division.

The National Institutes of Health (NIH) is the largest biomedical research center in the world. It's the research arm of the Public Health Service, U.S. Department of Health and Human Services. A helpful resource is CHID Online: The Combined Health Information Database. Website: www.chid.nih.gov
Among its institutes that conduct and support research on hepatitis viruses are the National Institute of Allergy and Infectious Diseases (NIAID) and the National Institute of Diabetes & Digestive & Kidney Diseases (NIDDK).

National Institute of Allergy and Infectious Diseases (NIAID)
The NIAID has the largest budget for research into viral hepatitis. For information on hepatitis B, write to:
NIAID Office of Communications
Building 31
Room 7A50
Bethesda, MD 20892
301-496-5717
Press releases, fact sheets, and other materials are available on the Internet via the NIAID home page: www.niaid.nih.gov

National Institute of Diabetes &
Digestive & Kidney Diseases (NIDDK)
For information on hepatitis B, write to:
National Digestive Diseases Information Clearinghouse (NDDIC)
2 Information Way
Bethesda, MD 20892-3570
Website: www.niddk.nih.gov
Email: nddic@info.niddk.nih.gov

Transplant Organizations and Agencies

Children's Liver Alliance
3835 Richmond Avenue
Box 190
Staten Island, NY 10312
Phone/Fax: 718-987-6200
Website: http://livertx.org
Email: livers4kids@earthlink.net

Transplant Recipient International Organization (TRIO)
Nationwide support group for patients and families
1000 16th St. NW
Suite 602
Washington, DC 20036-5705
1-800-TRIO-386
202-293-0980
Website: www.trioweb.org

United Network for Organ Sharing (UNOS)
1100 Boulders Parkway
Suite 500
P.O. Box 13770
Richmond, VA 23225-8770
804-330-8500
Patient information: 1-888-TX INFO1 (1-888-894-6361)
Website: www.unos.org

U.S. Department of Health and Human Services

Division of Transplantation
5600 Fishers Lane
Room 481
Rockville, MD 20857
301-443-7577
Website: www.hrsa.gov/osp/dot
Website: www.organdonor.gov

Note: Multiple Internet sites with information on hepatitis B exist. Although many have important information, we do not specifically endorse any of these sites although we have used resources from government-based websites in the production of this book.

Bibliography

Chapter 1

American Liver Foundation. 1996. *Hepatitis B.* New York: American Liver Foundation.

Bader, Teddy F. 1995. *Viral Hepatitis: Practical Evaluation and Treatment.* Seattle: Hogrefe & Huber.

Balkwill, Fran R. 1993. *DNA Is Here To Stay.* Mpls: Lerner Publishing Group.

Blumberg, Baruch S. 1997. *Hepatitis B Virus, the Vaccine, and the Control of Primary Cancer of the Liver.* National Academy of Sciences. 94:7121-7125.

Blumberg, Baruch S., Alton I. Sutnick, W. Thomas London, Irving Millman. 1972. *Australia Antigen and Hepatitis.* Cleveland: CRC Press.

Chan, H.L.Y., N.W.Y. Leung, M. Hussain, M.L. Wong, A.S.F. Lok. 2000. Hepatitis B e Antigen-Negative Chronic Hepatitis B in Hong Kong. *Hepatology.* 31:763-768.

De Franchis, R., G. Meucci, M. Vecchi, M. Tatarella, M. Colombo, E. Del Ninno, M.G. Rumi, M.F. Donato, G. Ronchi. 1993. The Natural History of Asymptomatic Hepatitis B Surface Antigen Carriers. *Annals of Internal Medicine.* 118:191-194.

Di Marco, V., O.L. Iacono, C. Camma, A. Vaccaro, M. Giunta, G. Martoran, P. Fuschi, P.L. Almasio, A. Craxi. 1999. The Long-Term Course of Chronic Hepatitis B. *Hepatology.* 30:257-264.

"Geographic Pattern of Hepatitis B Prevalence, 1997." 4 June 1998. *World Health Organization.* http://www.who.int/vaccines-surveillance/graphics/htmls/hepbprev.htm. 1 Aug. 2000.

"Global Status of Hepatitis B Immunisation Policy, as of March 2000." *World Health Organization.* http://www/who.int/vaccines-surveillance/graphics/htmls/hepb.htm. 1 Aug. 2000.

"Hepatitis B/Fact Sheet." Nov. 1998. *World Health Organization.* http://www.who.int/inf-fs/en/fact204.html. 1 Aug. 2000.

"Hepatitis B Vaccine-Fact Sheet." 2 Feb. 2000. *Centers for Disease Control and Prevention.* http://www.cdc.gov/ncidod/diseases/hepatitis/b/factvax.htm. 1 Aug. 2000.

Hepatitis B Foundation. 1995. *The Hepatitis B Story.* Warminster: Pennsylvania.

Hepatitis Foundation International. 1999. *Hepatitis B.* Cedar Grove: New Jersey.

Hoofnagle, Jay H. 1990. Posttransfusion Hepatitis B. *Transfusion.* Vol. 30 No. 5: 384-386.

Hoofnagle, J. H., D.A. Shafritz, H. Popper. 1987. Chronic Type B Hepatitis and the "Healthy" HBsAg Carrier State. *Hepatology.* Vol. 7, No. 4: 758-763.

Huo T-I., J-C. Wu, P-C. Lee, G-Y. Chau, W-Y. Lui, S-H. Tsay, L-T. Ting, F. Chang, S. Lee. 1998. Sero-Clearance of Hepatitis B Surface Antigen in Chronic Carriers Does Not Necessarily Imply a Good Prognosis. *Hepatology.* 28:2331-236.

Mandell, G.L., J.E. Bennett, R. Dolin, eds. 1995. *Principles and Practice of Infectious Diseases,* Vol.2. New York: Churchill Livingstone.

McMahon, B.J. July 1998. Chronic Carriers of Hepatitis B Virus Who Clear Hepatitis B Surface Antigen: Are They Really "off the Hook?" *Hepatology.* 265-267.

National Institutes of Health. 1997. Management of Hepatitis C. *NIH Consensus Statement 1997.* Mar 24-26; 15(3):1-41.

Radetsky, P. 1994. *The Invisible Invaders: Viruses and the Scientists Who Pursue Them.* Boston: Little, Brown and Co.

Schreiber, G.B., M.P. Busch, S.H. Kleinman, J.J. Korelitz. 1996. The Risk of Transfusion-Transmitted Viral Infections. *New England Journal of Medicine.* 334:1685-90.

Silverstein, Alvin, Virginia, Robert. 1994. *Hepatitis.* Springfield: Enslow Publishers.

Veres, Barbara. 2000. Discovery of the Hepatitis B Virus. *Hepatitis Magazine.* Sept./Oct., Vol. 2 No. 5: 8-9.

"Viral Hepatitis B-Fact Sheet." 5 July 2000. *Centers for Disease Control and Prevention.* http://www.cdc.gov/ncidod/diseases/hepatitis/b/index.htm. 1 Aug. 2000.

Villenueve, J-P, M. Desvrochers, C. Infante-Rivard, B. Willems, G. Raymond, M. Bourcier, J. Côté, G. Richer. 1994. A Long-term Follow-up Study of Asymptomatic Hepatitis B Surface Antigen-Positive Carriers in Montreal. *Gastroenterology*:106:1000-1005

Chapter 2

De Jongh, F.E., H.L.A. Janssen, R.A.De Man, W.C.J. Hop, S.W. Schalm, M.Van Blankenstein. 1992. Survival and Prognostic Indicators in Hepatitis B Surface Antigen-Positive Cirrhosis of the Liver. *Gastroenterology.* 103:1630-1635.

Hoofnagle, J.H. Aug. 2, 1990. Chronic Hepatitis B. *Hepatology.* Vol. 323, No. 5:337-339.

Lee, William M. 1997. Hepatitis B Virus Infection. *Medical Progress.* Vol. 337, No. 24:1733-45.

Shetty, K., Younossi, Z.M. 1998. Diagnostic Tests for Viral Hepatitis B and C. *Practical Gastroenterology.* 22(5):39-47.

Toshiyuki, M., F. Schödel, S. Iino, K. Koike, K. Yasuda, D. Peterson, D. R. Milich. 1994. Distinguishing Between Acute and Symptomatic Chronic Hepatitis B Virus Infection. *Gastroenterology.* 106:1006-1015.

Chapter 3

Alter, H. J., C. Conry-Cantilena, J. Melpolder, D. Tan, M. Van Raden, D. Herion, D. Lau, J. H. Hoofnagle. 1997. Hepatitis C in Asymptomatic Blood Donors. *Hepatology.* The National Institutes of Health Consensus Development Conference: Management of Hepatitis C. 26 (Suppl 1):29S-33S.

Boag, F. 1991. Hepatitis B: Heterosexual Transmission and Vaccination Strategies. *International Journal of STD & AIDS.* 2:318-324.

Castrone, L. 2 July 1996. Piercing and Tattooing, Body Language of 90s Worries Health Experts. *Rocky Mountain News.* 3D.

Galambos, John T. 1986. Transmission of Hepatitis B from Providers to Patients: How Big is the Risk? *Hepatology.* Vol. 6, No. 2:320-325.

"Government Urges Safer Needles." Federal Drug Administration. *FDA Consumer.* March–April 2000:2.

Harpaz, R., L. Von Seidlein, F. M. Averhoff, M.P. Tormey, S.D. Sinha, K. Kotsopoulou, S.B Lambert, B.H. Robertson, J.D. Cherry, C.N. Shapiro. 1996. Transmission of Hepatitis B Virus to Multiple Patients from a Surgeon Without Evidence of Inadequate Infection Control. *New England Journal of Medicine.* Vol. 334:549-54.

Hoyos, M., J.V. Sarrión, T. Péres-Castellanos, M. Prieto, M.L. Marty, V. Garrigues, J. Berenguer. 1989. Prospective Assessment of Donor Blood Screening for Antibody to Hepatitis B Core Antigen as a Means of Preventing Posttransfusion Non-A, Non-B, Hepatitis. *Hepatology.* 9:449-451.

Polish, L.B., C.N. Shapiro, F. Bauer, P. Klotz, P. Ginier, R.R. Roberto, M.S. Margolis, M.J. Alter. 1992. Nosocomial Transmission of Hepatitis B Virus Associated with the Use of a Spring-Loaded Finger-Stick Device. *New England Journal of Medicine.* 326: 721-5.

Kelen, G.D., G.B. Green, R.H. Purcell, D.W. Chan, B.F. Qaqish, K.T. Sivertson, T.C. Quinn. 1992. Hepatitis B and Hepatitis C in Emergency Department Patients. *New England Journal of Medicine.* 326:1399-404.

LaBrecque, D.R., J.M. Muhs, L.I. Lutwick, R.F. Woolson, W.R. Hierholzer. 1986. The Risk of Hepatitis B Transmission from Health Care Workers to Patients in a Hospital Setting – A Prospective Study. *Hepatology.* Vol. 6, No. 2:205-208.

Long, G.E., L.S. Rickman. 1994. Infectious Complications of Tattoos. *Clinical Infectious Diseases.* 18:610-9.

Minuk, G.Y., C.E. Bohme, T.J. Bowen, D.I. Hoar, S. Cassol, M.J. Gill, H. De C. Clarke. 1987. Efficacy of Commercial Condoms in the Prevention of Hepatitis B Virus Infection. *Gastroenterology.* 93:710-4.

"Needle Safety Jabs World's Attention." Hepatitis Foundation International. *Hepatitis Alert.* Summer 2000: 6.

Norman, J.E., G.W. Beebe, J.H. Hoofnagle, L.B. Seeff. 1993. Mortality Follow-up of the 1942 Epidemic of Hepatitis B in the U.S. Army. *Hepatology.* 18:790-797.

Scott, R.M., R. Snitbhan, W.H. Bancroft, H.J. Alter, M. Tingpalopong. July 1980. Experimental Transmission of Hepatitis B Virus by Semen and Saliva. *The Journal of Infectious Diseases.* Bol. 142, No. 1:67-71.

Seeff, L.B., G.W. Beebe, J.H. Hoofnagle, J.E. Norman, Z. Buskell-Bales, J.G. Waggoner, N. Kaplowitz, R.S. Koff, J.L. Petrini, E.R. Schiff, J. Shorey, M.M. Stanley. 1987. A Serologic Follow-Up of the 1942 Epidemic of Post-Vaccination Hepatitis in the United States Army. *New England Journal of Medicine.* 316:965-70.

"Someone You Know Has Hepatitis B. Are You In Danger?" 15 Aug. 2000. *Pkids.* http://www.pkids.org/someone_you_know.htm.

"Summary of Findings from the 1999 National Household Survey on Drug Abuse." 10 Oct. 2000. *Substance Abuse and Mental Health Services Administration.* http://www.samhsa.gov/oas/NHSDA/1999/Chapter2.htm.

"Testimony of Harold S. Margolis, M.D., Chief, Hepatitis Branch, Division of Viral and Rickettsial Diseases, National Center for Infectious Diseases, Centers for Disease Control and Prevention, Before the U.S. House of Representative Committee on Government Reform, Subcommittee on Criminal Justice, Drug

Policy, and Human Resources." 18 May 1999. *Centers for Disease Control.* http://www.cdc.gov/ncidod/diseases/hepatitis/margolis.htm. 1 Aug. 2000.

Tobe, Kazuo, K. Matsuura, T. Ogura, Y. Tsuo, Y. Iwasaki, M. Mizuno, K. Yamamoto, T. Higashi, T. Tsuji. 2000. Horizontal Transmission of Hepatitis B Virus Among Players of an American Football Team. *Archives of Internal Medicine.* 160:2541-2545.

Chapter 4

Damjanov, I., R.L. Moser , S. M. Katz, P. Lyons. Sept. 1980. Immune Complex Myositis Associated with Viral Hepatitis. *Human Pathology.* Vol. 11, No. 5: 478-481.

Guillevin, L., F. Lhote, P. Cohen, F. Sauvaget, B. Jarrousse, O. Lortholary, L-H, Noel, C. Trépo. 1995. Polyarteritis Nodosa Related to Hepatitis B Virus. *Medicine.* 74(5):238-253.

Hamilton, E. 1940, reprint 1989. *Mythology, Timeless Tales of Gods and Heroes.* Reprint. New York: Meridian.

Joven, J., C. Villabona, E. Vilella, L. Masana, R. Albertí, M. Vallés. 1990. Abnormalities of Lipoprotein Metabolism in Patients with the Nephrotic Syndrome. *New England Journal of Medicine.* 323:579-84.

Lai, K.N., P.K.T. Li, S.F. Lui, T.C. Au, J.S.L. Tam, K.L. Tong, F. Mac-M. Lai. 1991. Membranous Nephropathy Related to Hepatitis B Virus in Adults. *New England Journal of Medicine.* 324:1457-63,

Lisker-Melman, M., D. Webb, A.M. Di Bisceglie, C. Kassianides, P. Martin, V. Rustgi, J.G. Waggoner, Y. Park, J.H. Hoofnagle. 1989. Glomerulonephritis Caused by Chronic Hepatitis B Virus Infection: Treatment with Recombinant Human Alpha-Interferon. *Annals of Internal Medicine.* 111:479-483.

Lyons, A.S., J.R. Petrucelli, II. 1978. *Medicine, An Illustrated History.* New York: Harry N. Abrams.

McMahon, B.J., W.L. Heyward, D.W. Templin, D. Clement, A.P. Lanier. 1989. Hepatitis B-Associated Polyarteritis Nodosa in Alaskan Eskimos: Clinical and Epidemiologic Features and Long-Term Follow-up. *Hepatology.* 9(1): 97-101.

Neruda, Pablo. 1977. *Nuevas Odas Elementales, Cuarta Edicion.* Buenos Aires; Editorial Losada.

Scully, R.E., E.J. Mark, B. U. McNeely, eds. 1985. Case Records of the Massachusetts General Hospital (Case 36-1985). *New England Journal of Medicine.* 313(10): 622-630.

"Sculpture in Spain Salutes the 'Silent, Unselfish' Liver." *Austin-American Statesman.* 28 June 1987: A2.

Chapter 5

Angell, M., J.P. Kassirer. 1998. Alternative Medicine — The Risks of Untested and Unregulated Remedies. *New England Journal of Medicine.* 339:839-841.

Boigk, G., L. Stroedter, H. Herbst, J. Waldschmidt, E.O. Riecken, D. Schuppan. 1997. Silymarin Retards Collagen Accumulation in Early and Advanced Biliary Fibrosis Secondary to Complete Bile Duct Obliteration in Rats. *Hepatology.* 26:643-649.

Breidenbach, T.H., M.W. Hoffman, T.H. Becker, H. Schlitt, J. Klempnauer. 27 May 2000. Drug Interaction of St. John's Wort with Cyclosporine. *Lancet.* 355:1912.

Coppes, M.J., R.A. Anderson, R.M. Egeler, J.E.A. Wolff. 1998. Alternative Therapies for the Treatment of Childhood Cancer. *New England Journal of Medicine.* 339:846.

DiPaola, R.S., H. Zhang, G.H. Lambert, R. Meeker, E. Licitra, M.M. Rafi, B.T. Zhu, H. Spaulding, S. Goodin, M.B. Toledano, W.N. Hait, M.A. Gallo. 1998. Clinical and Biologic Activity of an Estrogenic Herbal Combination (PC-SPES) in Prostate Cancer. *New England Journal of Medicine.* 339:785-791.

Eisenberg, D.M. 1997. Advising Patients Who Seek Alternative Medical Therapies. *Annals of Internal Medicine.* 127:61-69.

Greenwald, J. 1998. "Herbal Healing." *Time,* 23 Nov., 60-69.

Gugliotta, Guy. "Supplements Aren't So Healthy." *Denver Post.* 19 March 2000: 5A.

Ko, R.J. 1998. Adulterants in Asian Patent Medicines. *New England Journal of Medicine.* 339:847.

Kurtzweil, Paula. 1998. An FDA Guide to Dietary Supplements. *FDA Consumer.* Vol.32 No.5:28-35.

Larrey, D., G. P. Pageaux. 1995. Hepatotoxicity of Herbal Remedies and Mushrooms. *Seminars in Liver Disease.* 15:183-188.

Marquis, Christopher. 2000. 90% of U.S. Diets Lacking, Feds Say. *Denver Post.* 28 May, 24A.

Munoz, S.J. 1991. Nutritional Therapies in Liver Disease. *Seminars in Liver Disease.* 11:278-291.

"NBJ's Fifth Annual Overview of the Nutrition Industry," *Nutrition Business Journal.* Vol.V No. 7/8 2000: 1, 3-7.

Nompleggi, D.J., H.L. Bonkovsky. 1994. Nutritional Supplementation in Chronic Liver Disease: An Analytical Review. *Hepatology.* 19:518-533.

"Q and A's on Dietary Guidelines for Americans, 2000." 3 June 2000, *Center for Nutrition Policy and Promotion.* 1 Sept. 2000.
  http://www.usda.gov/cnpp/Pubs/DG2000/Qa5-2.pdf.

"Research Funding Up for Alternative Medicine." Hepatitis Foundation International. *Hepatitis Alert.* Spring 2000, Vol. VI, No. 2: 6.

Schuppan, D., J.D. Jia, B. Brinkhaus, E.G. Hahn. 1999. Herbal Products for Liver Diseases: A Therapeutic Challenge for the New Millennium. *Hepatology.* 30:1099-1104.

Slifman, N.R., W.R. Obermeyer, S.M. Musser, W.A. Correll, S.M. Cichowicz, J.M. Betz, L.A. Love. 1998. Contamination of Botanical Dietary Supplements by Digitalis Lanata. *New England Journal of Medicine.* 339:806-811.

U.S. Department of Agriculture, U.S. Department of Health and Human Services. 1995. *Dietary Guidelines for Americans.* Fourth Edition. Washington.

Woolf, G.M., L.M. Petrovic, S.E. Rojter, S. Wainwright, F.G. Villamil, W.N. Katkov, P. Michieletti, I.R. Wanless, F.R. Stermitz, J.J. Beck, J. M. Vierling. 1994. Acute Hepatitis Associated with the Chinese Herbal Product Jin Bu Huan. *Annals of Internal Medicine.* 121:729-735.

Chapter 6

Anderson, Greg. 1993. *50 Essential Things to Do When the Doctor Says It's Cancer.* New York: Plume/Penguin.

Benson, Herbert with Marg Stark. 1996. *Timeless Healing, the Power and Biology of Belief.* New York: Scribner.

Benson, Herbert with Miriam Z. Klipper. 1975. *The Relaxation Response.* New York: Avon.

LeShan, Lawrence. 1994. *Cancer As a Turning Point.* New York: Plume/Penguin.

Moyers, Bill. 1993. *Healing and the Mind.* New York: Doubleday.

Spiegel, David, M.D. 1993. *Living Beyond Limits.* New York: Random House.

Topf, Linda Noble with Hal Z. Bennett. 1995. *You Are Not Your Illness.* New York: Fireside.

Chapter 7

Beam, Jr., Burton T. and Kenn B. Tacchino. Jan. 1997. *The Health Insurance Portability and Accountability Act of 1996.* Journal of the American Society of CLU & ChFC. 14+.

Health Care Financing Administration. Sept. 2000. *Medicare & You 2001.* Publication No. HCFA-10050. Washington: U.S. Government Printing Office.

Health Care Financing Administration. March 2000. *2000 Guide to Health Insurance for People with Medicare.* Publication No. HCFA-02110. Washington: U.S. Government Printing Office.

Hepatitis B Foundation. August 2000. *HFB Drug Watch: Compounds in Development for Chronic Hepatitis B.* Warminster, Pennsylvania.

Jehle, Faustin F. July 1998. *The Complete and Easy Guide to Social Security, Healthcare Rights & Government Benefits.* Boca Raton: Emerson-Adams Press.

Social Security Administration. July 1999. *Social Security Supplemental Security Income.* SSA Publication No. 05-11000. Washington.

Social Security Administration. Sept. 1995. *Social Security Disability Programs Can Help.* SSA Publication No. 05-10057. Washington.

Social Security Administration. Aug. 2000. *Social Security Disability Benefits.* SSA Publication No. 05-10029. Washington.

U.S. Department of Labor Employment Standards Administration, Wage and Hour Division. Dec. 1996. Publication 1421. *Compliance Guide to the Family and Medical Leave Act.* Washington: U.S. Government Printing Office.

U.S. Department of Labor Employment Standards Administration, Wage and Hour Division. April 1995. WH Publication 1419. Federal Regulations Part 825. *The Family and Medical Leave Act of 1993.* Washington: U.S. Government Printing Office.

U.S. Department of Labor Employment Standards Administration, Wage and Hour Division. June 1993. WH Publication 1420. *Your Rights Under the Family and Medical Leave Act of 1993.* Washington: U.S. Government Printing Office.

U.S. Department of Labor Program. 1993. *The Family and Medical Leave Act of 1993.* Highlights Fact Sheet No. ESA 93-2. Washington: U.S. Government Printing Office.

U.S. Equal Employment Opportunity Commission, U.S. Department of Justice,

Civil Rights Division. 1992. *The Americans with Disabilities Act, Questions and Answers.* Washington.

U.S. Equal Employment Opportunity Commission. 1991. *The Americans With Disabilities Act.* Washington.

United Network for Organ Sharing (UNOS). 1997. *What Every Patient Needs to Know.*

Chapter 8

Allen, M.I., M. Deslauriers, C.W. Andrews, G.A. Tipples, K-A Walters, D.L.J. Tyrrell, N. Brown, for the Lamivudine Clinical Investigation Group, and L.D. Condreay. 1998. Identification and Characterization of Mutations in Hepatitis B Virus Resistant to Lamivudine. *Hepatology.* 27:1670-1677.

Ascherio, A., S.M. Zhang, M.A. Hernan, M.J. Olek, P.M. Coplan, K. Brodovicz, A.M Walker. 2001. Hepatitis B Vaccination and the Risk of Multiple Sclerosis. *New England Journal of Medicine.* 344:327-32.

Benhamou, Y. C. Katlama, F. Lunel, A. Coutellier, E. Dohin, N. Hamm, R. Tubiana, S. Herson, T. Poynard, P. Opolon. 1996. Effects of Lamivudine on Replication of Hepatitis B Virus in HIV-Infected Men. *Annals of Internal Medicine.* 125:705-712.

Bloom, B.S., A.L. Hillman, A.M. Fendrick, J.S. Schwartz. 1993. A Reappraisal of Hepatitis B Virus Vaccination Strategies Using Cost-Effectiveness Analysis. *Annals of Internal Medicine.* 118:298-306.

Blumberg, B. July 1997. *Hepatitis B Virus, the Vaccine, and the Control of Primary Cancer of the Liver.* Procedings of the National Academy of Sciences. Vol. 94:7121-7125.

Bonkovsky, H.L., B.F. Banner, A.L. Rothman. 1997. Iron and Chronic Viral Hepatitis. *Hepatology.* 25:759-767.

Brook, M.G., P. Karayiannis, H.C. Thomas. 1989. Which Patients with Chronic Hepatitis B Virus Infection Will Respond to Alpha-Interferon Therapy? A Statistical Analysis of Predictive Factors. *Hepatology.* Vol. 10, No. 5:761-763.

Brunetto, M.R., M. Giarin, G. Saracco, F. Oliveri, P. Calvo, G. Capra, A. Randone, M.L. Abate, P. Manzini, M. Capalbo, P. Piantino, G. Verme, F. Bonino. 1993. Hepatitis B Virus Unable to Secrete e Antigen and Response to Interferon in Chronic Hepatitis B. *Gastroenterology.* 105:845-850.

Chang, M-H., C-J. Chen, M-S. Lai, H-M. Hsu, T-C. Wu, M-S. Kong, D-C. Liang, W-Y. Shau, D-S. Chen, for the Taiwan Childhood Hepatoma Study Group. 1997. Universal Hepatitis B Vaccination in Taiwan and the Incidence of Hepatocellular Carcinoma in Children. *New England Journal of Medicine.* 336:1855-9.

Chayama, K.Y. Suzuki, M. Kobayashi, M. Kobayashi, A. Tsubota, M. Hashimoto, Y. Miyano, H. Koike, M. Kobayashi, I. Koida, Y. Arase, S. Saitoh, N. Murashima, K. Ikeda, H. Kumada. 1998. Emergence and Takeover of YMDD Motif Mutant Hepatitis B Virus During Long-Term Lamivudine Therapy and Re-takeover by Wild Type After Cessation of Therapy. *Hepatology.* 27:1711-1716.

Confavreux, C., S. Suissa, P. Saddier, V. Bourdes, S. Vukusic, for the Vaccines in Multiple Sclerosis Study Group. 2001. Vaccinations and the Risk of Relapse in Multiple Sclerosis. *New England Journal of Medicine.* 344:319-26.

Cotonat, T., J.A. Quiroga, J.M. López-Alcorocho, R. Clouet, M. Pardo, F. Manzarbeitia, V. Carreño. 2000. Pilot Study of Combination Therapy With Ribavirin and Interferon Alfa for the Retreatment of Chronic Hepatitis B e Antibody-Positive patients. *Hepatology*. 31:502-506.

Dienstag, J.L., E.R. Schiff, T.L. Wright, R. P. Perrillo, H-W. L. Hann, Z. Goodman, L. Crowther, L.D. Condreay, M. Woessner, M. Rubin, N.A. Brown, for the U.S. Lamivudine Investigator Group. 1999. Lamivudine As Initial Treatment For Chronic Hepatitis B In the United States. *New England Journal of Medicine*. 341:1256-63.

Dienstag, J.L., E.R. Schiff, M. Mitchell, D.E. Casey, Jr., N. Gitlin, T. Lissoos, L.D. Gelb, L. Condreay, L. Crowther, M. Rubin, N. Brown. 1999. Extended Lamivudine Retreatment for Chronic Hepatitis B: Maintenance of Viral Suppression After Discontinuation of Therapy. *Hepatology*. 30:1082-1087.

Dienstag, J.L., R.P. Perrillo, E.R. Schiff, M. Bartholomew, C. Vicary, M. Rubin. 1995. A Preliminary Trial of Lamivudine For Chronic Hepatitis B Infection. *New England Journal of Medicine*. 333:1657-61.

Dusheiko, G.M., J.A. Roberts. 1995. Treatment of Chronic Type B and C Hepatitis with Interferon Alfa: an Economic Appraisal. *Hepatology*. 22:1863-1873.

Fattovich, G., G. Giustina, G. Realdi, R. Corrocher, S.W. Schalm, and the European Concerted Action on Viral Hepatitis (Eurohep). 1997. Long-Term Outcome of Hepatitis B e Antigen-Positive Patients With Compensated Cirrhosis Treated with Interferon Alfa. *Hepatology*. 26:1338-1342.

Fontana, R.J., A.S.F. Lok. 1997. Combination Therapy for Chronic Hepatitis B. *Hepatology*. Vol. 26, No. 1:234-237.

Gish, R.G., J.Y.N. Lau, L. Brooks, J.W.S. Fang, S.L. Steady, J.C. Imperial, R. Garcia-Kennedy, C.O. Esquivel, E.B. Keeffe. 1996. Ganciclovir Treatment of Hepatitis B Virus Infection in Liver Transplant Recipients. *Hepatology*. 23:1-7.

Hadziyannis S.J., G.V. Papatheodoridis, E. Dimou, A. Laras, C. Papaioannou. 2000. Efficacy of Long-Term Lamivudine Monotherapy in Patients With Hepatitis B e Antigen-Negative Chronic Hepatitis B. *Hepatology*. 32:847-851.

"Hepatitis B Vaccine." 29 Sept. 2000. *Centers for Disease Control and Prevention*. http://www.cdc.gov/ncidod/diseases/hepatitis/b/faqbvax.htm.   29   Dec. 2000.

"Hepatitis B Vaccine, What You Need to Know, Vaccine Information Statement (Interim)." 9 Aug. 2000. *Centers for Disease Control and Prevention*. http://www.cdc.gov/nip/publications/vis/vis-hep-b.pdf. 29 Dec. 2000.

Honkoop, P., R.A. De Man, H.G.M. Niesters, P.E. Zondervan, S.W. Schalm. 2000. Acute Exacerbation of Chronic Hepatitis B Virus Infection After Withdrawal of Lamivudine Therapy. *Hepatology*. Vol.32, No. 3:635-639.

Hoofnagle, J.H., A.M. Di Bisceglie, J.G. Waggoner, Y. Park. 1993. Interferon Alfa for Patients With Clinically Apparent Cirrhosis Due to Chronic Hepatitis B. *Gastroenterology*. 104:1116-1121.

Huang, L-M., B-L. Chiang, C-Y. Lee, P-I. Lee, W-K. Chi, M-H. Chang. 1999. Long-Term Response to Hepatitis B Vaccination and Response to Booster in Children Born to Mothers with Hepatitis B e Antigen. *Hepatology*. 29:954-959.

Hunt, C.M. , J.M. McGill, M.I. Allen, L.D. Condreay. May 2000. Clinical Relevance of Hepatitis B Viral Mutations. *Hepatology*. 31:1037-1044.

Janssen, H.L.A., G. Gerken, V. Carreño, P. Marcellin, N.V. Naoumov, A. Craxi, H. Ring-Larsen, G. Kitis, J. van Hattum, R.A. De Vries, P.P. Michielsen, F.J.W. Ten Kate, W.C.J. Hop, R.A. Heijtink, P. Honkoop, S.W. Schalm, and the European Concerted Action on Viral Hepatitis (EUROHEP). 1999. Interferon Alfa for Chronic Hepatitis B Infection: Increased Efficacy of Prolonged Treatment. *Hepatology*. 30:238-243.

Jurim, O., P. Martin, D.J. Winston, C. Shackleton, C. Holt, J. Feller, M. Csete, A. Shaked, D. Imagawa, K. Olthoff, J.Y.N. Lau, R.W. Busuttil. 1996. Failure of Ganciclovir Prophylaxis to Prevent Allograft Reinfection Following Orthotopic Liver Transplantation for Chronic Hepatitis B Infection. *Liver Transplantation and Surgery*. Vol. 2, No. 5 (Sept.):370-374.

Koff, R.S., L.B. Seeff. 1995. Economic Modeling of Treatment in Chronic Hepatitis B and Chronic Hepatitis C: Promises and Limitations. *Hepatology*. 22:1880-82.

Korenman, J., B. Baker, J. Waggoner, J.E. Everhart, A.M. Di Bisceglie, J.H. Hoofnagle. 1991. Long-Term Remission of Chronic Hepatitis B after Alpha-Interferon Therapy. *Annals of Internal Medicine*. 114:629-634.

Krüger, M., H.L. Tillmann, C. Trautwein, U. Bode, K. Oldhafer, H. Maschek, K.H.W. Böker, C.E. Broelsch, R. Pichlmayr, M.P. Manns. 1996. Famciclovir Treatment of Hepatitis B Virus Recurrence After Liver Transplantation: A Pilot Study. *Liver Transplantation and Surgery*. Vol.2, No.4:253-262.

Kuhns, M., A. McNamara, A. Mason, C. Campbell, R. Perrillo. 1992. Serum and Liver Hepatitis B Virus DNA in Chronic Hepatitis B After Sustained Loss of Surface Antigen. *Gastroenterology*. 103:1649-1656.

Lai, C-L., R-N. Chien, N.W.Y. Leung, T-T. Chang, R. Guan, D-I. Tai, K-Y Ng, P-C. Wu, J.C. Dent, J. Barber, S.L. Stephenson, D. F. Gray, for the Asia Hepatitis Lamivudine Study Group. 1998. A One-Year Trial Of Lamivudine For Chronic Hepatitis B. *New England Journal of Medicine*. 339:61-8.

Lai, C-L., B.C-Y. Wong, E-K. Yeoh, W-L. Lim, W-K. Chang, H-J. Lin. 1993. Five-year Follow-up of a Prospective Randomized Trial of Hepatitis B Recombinant DNA Yeast Vaccine in Children: Immunogenicity and Anamnestic Responses. *Hepatology*. 18:763-767.

Lampertico, P., E. Del Ninno, A. Manzin, M.F. Donato, M.G. Rumi, G. Lunghi, A. Morabito, M. Clementi, M.Colombo. 1997. A Randomized, Controlled Trial of a 24-Month Course of Interferon Alfa 2b in Patients with Chronic Hepatitis B Who Had Hepatitis B Virus DNA without Hepatitis B e Antigen in Serum. *Hepatology*. 26:1621-1625.

Lau, D.T-Y., M.F. Khokhar, E. Doo, M.G. Ghany, D. Herion, Y. Park, D.E. Kleiner, P. Schmid, L.D. Condreay, J. Gauthier, M.C. Kuhns, T.J. Liang, J.H. Hoofnagle. 2000. Long-Term Therapy of Chronic Hepatitis B With Lamivudine. *Hepatology*. 32:828-834.

Lau, D. T-Y., E. Doo, Y. Park, D.E. Kleiner, P. Schmid, M.C. Kuhns, J.H. Hoofnagle. 1999. Lamivudine for Chronic Delta Hepatitis. *Hepatology*. 30:546-549.

Lau, D. T-Y., J. Everhart, D. E. Kleiner, Y. Park, J.Vergalla, P. Schmid, J.H. Hoofnagle.

1997. Long-term Follow-up of Patients With Chronic Hepatitis B Treated With Interferon Alfa. *Gastroenterology*. 113:1660-1667.

Liaw, Y-F., N.W.Y. Leung, T-T. Chang, R. Guan, D-I. Tai, K-Y. Ng, R-N. Chien, J. Dent, L. Roman, S. Edmundson, C-L. Lai, for the Asia Hepatitis Lamivudine Study Group. 2000. Effects of Extended Lamivudine Therapy in Asian Patients With Chronic Hepatitis B. *Gastroenterology*. 119:172-180.

Liaw, Y-F., R-N. Chien, C-T. Yeh, S-L. Tsai, C-M. Chu. 1999. Acute Exacerbation and Hepatitis B Virus Clearance After Emergence of YMDD Motif Mutation During Lamivudine Thereapy. *Hepatology*. 30:567-572.

Lin, S-M., I-S. Sheen, R-N. Chien, C-M. Chu, Y-F. Liaw. 1999. Long-Term Beneficial Effect of Interferon Therapy in Patients With Chronic Hepatitis B Virus Infection. *Hepatology*. 29:971-975.

Lok, A.S.F. July 2000. Lamivudine therapy for Chronic Hepatitis B: Is Longer Duration of Treatment Better? *Gastroenterology*. Vol. 119, No. 1:263-266.

Lok, A.S.F. 1993. Antiviral Therapy of the Asian Patient with Chronic Hepatitis B. *Seminars In Liver Disease*. Vol. 13, No. 4: 360-366.

Lok, A.S.F., H-T. Chung, V.W.S. Liu, O.C.K. Ma. 1993. Long-Term Follow-up of Chronic Hepatitis B Patients Treated With Interferon Alfa. *Gastroenterology*. 105:1833-1838.

Lok, A.S.F., P-C. Wu, C-L. Lai, J.Y.N. Lau, E.K.Y. Leung, L.S.K. Wong, O.C.K. Ma, I.J. Lauder, C.P.L. Ng, H-T. Chung. 1992. A Controlled Trial of Interferon With or Without Prednisone Priming for Chronic Hepatitis B. *Gastroenterology*. 102:2091-2097.

Lok, A.S.F., O.C.K. Ma, J.Y.N. Lau. 1991. Interferon Alfa Therapy in Patients With Chronic Hepatitis B Virus Infection, Effects on Hepatitis B Virus DNA in the Liver. *Gastroenterology*. 100:756-761.

Malik, A.H., W. M. Lee. 2000. Chronic Hepatitis B Virus Infection: Treatment Strategies for the Next Millennium. *Annals of Internal Medicine*. 132:723-731.

Malik, A.H., W.M.Lee. 1999. Hepatitis B Therapy: The Plot Thickens. *Hepatology*. Vol. 30, No. 2:579-581.

Nevens, F., J. Main, P. Honkoop, D.L. Tyrrell, J. Barber, M.T. Sullivan, J. Fevery. R.A. De Man, H.C. Thomas. 1997. Lamivudine Therapy for Chronic Hepatitis B: A Six-Month Randomized Dose-Ranging Study. *Gastroenterology*. 113:1258-1263.

Niederau, C., T. Heintges, S. Lange, G. Goldmann, C.M. Niederau, L. Mohr, D. Häussinger. 1996. Long-Term Follow-Up Of HBeAg-Positive Patients Treated With Interferon Alfa For Chronic Hepatitis B. *New England Journal of Medicine*. 334:1422-7.

Omata, M. 1998. Treatment of Chronic Hepatitis B Infection. *New England Journal of Medicine*. Vol. 339, No. 2: 114-115.

Perrillo, R., E. Schiff, E. Yoshida, A. Statler, K. Hirsch, T. Wright, K. Gutfreund, P. Lamy, A. Murray. 2000. Adefovir Dipivoxil for the Treatment of Lamivudine-Resistant Hepatitis B Mutants. *Hepatology*. 32:129-134.

Perrillo, R.P., C. Tamburro, F. Regenstein, L. Balart, H. Bodenheimer, M. Silva, E. Schiff, C. Bodicky, B. Miller, C. Denham, C. Brodeur, K. Roach, J. Albrecht. 1995. Low-Dose, Titratable Interferon Alfa in Decompensated Liver Disease

Caused by Chronic Infection With Hepatitis B Virus. *Gastroenterology.* 109:908–916.

Perrillo, R.P. April 1993. Interferon in the Management of Chronic Hepatitis B. *Digestive Diseases and Sciences.* Vol. 38, No. 4:577–593.

Perrillo, R.P., E.M. Brunt. 1991. Hepatic Histologic and Immunohistochemical Changes in Chronic Hepatitis B after Prolonged Clearance of Hepatitis B e Antigen and Hepatitis B Surface Antigen. *Annals of Internal Medicine.* 115:113–115.

Perrillo, R.P. 1990. Factors Influencing Response to Interferon in Chronic Hepatitis B: Implications for Asian and Western Populations. *Hepatology.* Vol. 12, No. 6:1433–1435.

Perrillo, R.P., E.R. Schiff, G.L. Davis, H.C. Bodenheimer, Jr., K. Lindsay, J. Payne, J.L. Dienstag, C. O'Brien, C. Tamburro, I.M. Jacobson, R. Sampliner, D. Feit, J. Lefkowitch, M. Kuhns, C. Meschievitz, B. Sanghvi, J. Albrecht, A. Gibas, and the Hepatitis Interventional Therapy Group. 1990. A Randomized, Controlled Trial Of Interferon Alfa-2b Alone And After Prednisone Withdrawal For The Treatment Of Chronic Hepatitis B. *New England Journal of Medicine.* 323:295–301.

Perrillo, R.P., F.G. Regenstein, M.G. Peters, K. DeSchryver-Kecskemeti, C.J. Bodicky, C.R. Campbell, M.C. Kuhns. 1988. Prednisone Withdrawal Followed by Recombinant Alpha Interferon in the Treatment of Chronic Type B Hepatitis. *Annals of Internal Medicine.* 109:95–100.

Richman, D.D., 2000. The Impact of Drug Resistance on the Effectiveness of Chemotherapy for Chronic Hepatitis B. *Hepatology.* Vol. 32, No. 4:866–867.

Schaffner, W., P. Gardner. 1993. Hepatitis B Immunization Strategies: Expanding the Target. *Annals of Internal Medicine.* 118:308–309.

Singh, N., T. Gayowski, C.F. Wannstedt, M.W. Wagener, I.R. Marino. 1997. Pretransplant Famciclovir As Prophylaxis For Hepatitis B Virus Recurrence After Liver Transplantation. *Transplantation.* Vol. 63, No. 10:1415–1419.

Snyder, Michael A. Sept./Oct. 2000. Research Yields Major Advances in Eradication of HBV – R. Palmer Beasley, M.D.: Researcher and Humanitarian. *Hepatitis.* Vol. 2 No. 5:18–20.

Song, B–C., D.J. Suh, H.C. Lee, Y–H. Chung, Y.S. Lee. 2000. Hepatitis B e Antigen Seroconversion After Lamivudine Therapy is Not Durable in Patients With Chronic Hepatitis B in Korea. *Hepatology.* 32:803–806.

Szmuness, W., C.E. Stevens, E.J. Harley, E.A. Zang, W.R. Oleszko, D.C. William, R. Sadovsky, J..M. Morrison, A. Kellner. 1980. Hepatitis B Vaccine, Demonstration of Efficacy in a Controlled Clinical Trial in a High-Risk Population in the United States. *New England Journal of Medicine.* 303:833–41.

Tassopoulos, N.C., R. Volpes, G. Pastore, J. Heathcote, M. Buti, R.D. Goldin, S. Hawley, J. Barber, L. Condreay, D.F. Gray, and the Lamivudine Precore Mutant Study Group. 1999. Efficacy of Lamivudine in Patients With Hepatitis B e Antigen-Negative/Hepatitis B Virus DNA-Positive (Precore Mutant) Chronic Hepatitis B. *Hepatology.* 29:889–896.

Torresi, J., S. Locarnini. 2000. Antiviral Chemotherapy for the Treatment of Hepatitis B Virus Infections. *Gastroenterology.* 118:S83–S103.

Villeneuve, J–P., L.D. Condreay, B. Willems, G Pomier-Layrargues, D. Fenyves, M.

Bilodeau, R. Leduc, K. Peltekian, F. Wong, M. Margulies, E.J. Heathcote. 2000. Lamivudine Treatment for Decompensated Cirrhosis Resulting From Chronic Hepatitis B. *Hepatology.* 31:207-210.

Wong, D.K.H., C. Yim, C.D. Naylor, E. Chen, M. Sherman, S. Vas, I.R. Wanless, S. Read, H. Li, E. J. Heathcote. 1995. Interferon Alfa Treatment of Chronic Hepatitis B: Randomized Trial in a Predominantly Homosexual Male Population. *Gastroenterology.* 108:165-171.

Wong, D.K.H., A.M. Cheung, K. O'Rourke, C.D. Naylor, A.S. Detsky, J. Heathcote. 1993. Effect of Alpha-Interferon Treatment in Patients with Hepatitis B e Antigen-Positive Chronic Hepatitis B, A Meta-Analysis. *Annals of Internal Medicine.* 119:312-323.

Wong, J.B., R.S. Koff, F. Tinè, S.G. Pauker. 1995. Cost-effectiveness of Interferon-Alfa2b Treatment for Hepatitis B e Antigen-Positive Chronic Hepatitis B. *Annals of Internal Medicine.* 122:664-675.

Woolf, G.M., L.M. Petrovic, S.E. Rojter, S. Wainwright, F.G. Villamil, W.N. Katkov, P. Michieletti, I.R. Wanless, F.R. Stermitz, J.J. Beck, J.M. Vierling. 1994. Acute Hepatitis Associated with the Chinese Herbal Product Jin Bu Huan. *Annals of Internal Medicine.* 121:729-735.

Xiong, X. C. Flores, H. Yang, J.J. Toole, C.S. Gibbs. 1998. Mutations in Hepatitis B DNA Polymerase Associated With Resistance to Lamivudine Do Not Confer Resistance to Adefovir *In Vitro. Hepatology.* 28:1669-1673.

Chapter 9

Ben-Ari, Z., D. Shmueli, E. Mor, Z. Shapira, R. Tur-Kaspa. 1997. Beneficial Effect Of Lamivudine In Recurrent Hepatitis B After Liver Transplantation. *Transplantation.* Vol. 63, No. 3:393-396

Benner, K.G., R.G. Lee, E.B. Keeffe, R.R. Lopez, A.W. Sasaki, C.W. Pinson. 1992. Fibrosing Cytolytic Liver Failure Secondary to Recurrent Hepatitis B After Liver Transplantation. *Gastroenterology.* 103:1307-1312.

Chalasani, N., G. Smallwood, J. Halcomb, M.W. Fried, T.D. Boyer. 1998. Is Vaccination Against Hepatitis B Infection Indicated in Patients Waiting for or After Orthotopic Liver Transplantation? *Liver Transplantation and Surgery.* Vol. 4, No. 2 (March):128-132.

Chan, T-M., P-C. Wu, F-K. Li, C-L. Lai, I.K.P. Cheng, K-N. Lai. 1998. Treatment of Fibrosing Cholestatic Hepatitis With Lamivudine. *Gastroenterology.* 115:177-181.

Dickson, R.C. 1998. Management of Posttransplantation Viral Hepatitis – Hepatitis B. *Liver Transplantation and Surgery.* Vol. 4, No. 5, Suppl. 1(Sept.): 573-578.

Eason, J.D., R.B. Freeman, Jr., R.J. Rohrer, W.D. Lewis, R. Jenkins, J. Dienstag, A.B. Cosimi. 1994. Should Liver Transplantation Be Performed For Patients With Hepatitis B? *Transplantation.* Vol. 57, No. 11:1588-1593.

Ghany, M.G., B. Ayola, F.G. Villamil, R.G. Gish, S. Rojter, J.M. Vierling, A.S.F. Lok. 1998. Hepatitis B Virus S Mutants in Liver Transplant Recipients Who Were Reinfected Despite Hepatitis B Immune Globulin Prophylaxis. *Hepatology.* 27:213-222.

Ho, B.M., S.K. So, C.O. Esquivel, E.B. Keeffe. 1997. Liver Transplantation in Asian Patients With Chronic Hepatitis B. *Hepatology.* 25:223-225.

Kitay-Cohen, Y., Z. Ben-Ari, R. Tur-Kaspa, H. Fainguelernt, M. Lishner. 2000. Extension Of Transplantation Free Time By Lamivudine In Patients with Hepatitis B-Induced Decompensated Cirrhosis. *Transplantation.* Vol. 69, No. 11:2382-2383.

Lucey, M.R. 1994. Hepatitis B Infection and Liver Transplantation: The Art of the Possible. *Hepatology.* 19:245-247.

Malkan, G., M.S. Cattral, A. Humar, H. A. Asghar, P.D. Greig, A. W. Hemming, G.A. Levy, L.B. Lilly. 2000. Lamivudine For Hepatitis B In Liver Transplantation. *Transplantation.* Vol. 69, No. 7:1403-1407.

Marinos, G., S. Rossol, P. Carucci, P.Y.N. Wong, P. Donaldson, M.J. Hussain, D. Vergani, B.C. Portmann, R. Williams, N. V. Naoumov. 2000. Immunopathogenesis Of Hepatitis B Virus Recurrence After Liver Transplantation. *Transplantation.* Vol. 69, No. 4:559-568.

Markowitz, J.S., P. Martin, A.J. Conrad, J.F. Markmann, P. Seu, H. Yersiz, J.A. Goss, P. Schmidt, A. Pakrasi, L. Artinian, N.G.B. Murray, D.K. Imagawa, C. Holt, L.I. Goldstein, R. Stribling, R.W. Busuttil. 1998. Prophylaxis Against Hepatitis B Recurrence Following Liver Transplantation Using Combination Lamivudine and Hepatitis B Immune Globulin. *Hepatology.* 28:585-589.

McGory, R.W., M.B. Ishitani, W.M. Oliveira, W.C. Stevenson, C.S. McCullough, R.C. Dickson, S.H. Caldwell, T.L. Pruett. 1996. Improved Outcome of Orthotopic Liver Transplantation For Chronic Hepatitis B Cirrhosis with Aggressive Passive Immunization. *Transplantation.* Vol. 61, No. 9:1358-1364.

Mutimer, D., G. Dusheiko, C. Barrett, L. Grellier, M. Ahmed, G. Anschuetz, A. Burroughs, S.. Hubscher, A.P. Dhillon, K. Rolles, E. Elias. 2000. Lamivudine Without HBIG For Prevention Of Graft Reinfection By Hepatitis B: Long-Term Follow-Up. *Transplantation.* Vol. 70, No. 5:809-815.

Naumann, U., U. Protzer-Knolle, T. Berg, K. Leder, H. Lobeck, W-O. Bechstein, G. Gerken, U. Hopf, P. Neuhaus. 1997. A Pretransplant Infection with Precore Mutants of Hepatitis B Virus Does Not Influence the Outcome of Orthotopic Liver Transplantation in Patients on High Dose Anti-Hepatitis B Virus Surface Antigen Immunoprophylaxis. *Hepatology.* 26:478-484.

Nery, J.R., D. Weppler, M. Rodriguez, P. Ruiz, E.R. Schiff, A.G. Tzakis. 1998. Efficacy Of Lamivudine In Controlling Hepatitis B Virus Recurrence After Liver Transplantation. *Transplantation.* Vol. 65, No. 12:1615-1621.

Perrillo, R., J. Rakela, J. Dienstag, G. Levy, P. Martin, T. Wright, S. Caldwell, E. Schiff, R. Gish, J.P. Villeneuve, G. Farr, F. Anschuetz, L. Crowther, N. Brown, and the Lamivudine Transplant Group. 1999. Multicenter Study of Lamivudine Therapy for Hepatitis B After Liver Transplantation. *Hepatology.* 29:1581-1586.

Poterucha, J.J., R.H. Wiesner. 1997. Liver Transplantation and Hepatitis B. *Annals of Internal Medicine.* 126:805-807.

Protzer-Knolle, U., U. Naumann, R. Bartenschlager, T. Berg, U. Hopf, K-H. Meyer zum Buschenfelde, P. Neuhaus, G. Gerken. 1998. Hepatitis B Virus With Antigenically Altered Hepatitis B Surface Antigen Is Selected by High-Dose Hepatitis B Immune Globulin After Liver Transplantation. *Hepatology.* 27:254-263.

Sanchez-Fueyo, A., A. Rimola, L. Grande, J. Costa, A. Mas, M. Navasa, I. Cirera, J.M. Sanchez-Tapias, J. Rodes. 2000. Hepatitis B Immunoglobulin Discontinuation

Followed by Hepatitis B Virus Vaccination: A New Strategy in the Prophylaxis of Hepatitis B Virus Recurrence After Liver Transplantation. *Hepatology.* 31:496-501.

Samuel, D., R. Muller, G. Alexander, L. Fassati, B. Ducot, J-P. Benhamou, H. Bismuth, and the Investigators of the European Concerted Action on Viral Hepatitis Study. 1993. Liver Transplantation in European Patients with the Hepatitis B Surface Antigen. *New England Journal of Medicine.* 329:1842-7.

Terrault, N.A., C.C. Holland, L. Ferrell, J.A. Hahn, J.R. Lake, J.P. Roberts, N.L. Ascher, T.L. Wright. 1996. Interferon Alfa for Recurrent Hepatitis B Infection After Liver Transplantation. *Liver Transplantation and Surgery.* Vol. 2, No. 2 (March):132-138.

Terrault, N.A., S. Zhou, C. Combs, J.A. Hahn, J.R. Lake, J.P. Roberts, N.L. Ascher, T.L. Wright. 1996. Prophylaxis in Liver Transplant Recipients Using a Fixed Dosing Schedule of Hepatitis B Immunoglobulin. *Hepatology.* 24:1327-1333.

Vierling, J.M., L.W. Teperman, A.P. Brownstein. December 1998. Hepatitis B: An Appropriate Indication for Liver Transplantation. *Results and Recommendations of a Hepatitis B Liver Transplant Symposium Sponsored by the American Liver Foundation.* 1-10.

Yao, F.Y., R.W. Osorio, J.P. Roberts, F.F. Poordad, M.N. Briceno, R. Garcia-Kennedy, R.R. Gish. 1999. Intramuscular Hepatitis B Immune Globulin Combined With Lamivudine for Prophylaxis Against Hepatitis B Recurrence After Liver Transplantation. *Liver Transplantation and Surgery.* Vol. 5, No. 6 (Nov.):491-496.

Chapter 10

Achkar, J-P., V. Araya, R.L. Baron, J.W. Marsh, I. Dvorchik, J. Rakela. 1998. Undetected Hepatocellular Carcinoma: Clinical Features and Outcome After Liver Transplantation. *Liver Transplantation and Surgery.* Vol. 4, No. 6 (Nov.):477-482.

Beasley, P.R., C-C. Lin, L-Y. Hwang, C-S. Chien. 1981. Hepatocellular Carcinoma and Hepatitis B Virus. *Lancet.* 2:1129-1133.

Bruix, J. 1997. Treatment of Hepatocellular Carcinoma. *Hepatology.* 25:259-261.

Chang, M-H., C-J. Chen, M-S. Lai, H-M. Hsu, T-C. Wu, M-S. Kong, D-C. Liang, W-Y. Shau, D-S. Chen, for the Taiwan Childhood Hepatoma Study Group. 1997. Universal Hepatitis B Vaccination in Taiwan and the Incidence of Hepatocellular Carcinoma in Children. *New England Journal of Medicine.* 336:1855-1859.

Collier, J., M. Sherman. 1998. Screening for Hepatocellular Carcinoma. *Hepatology.* 27:273-278.

Di Bisceglie, A.M., R.L. Carithers, Jr., G.J. Gores. 1998. Hepatocellular Carcinoma. *Hepatology.* Vol. 28, No. 4:1161-1165.

Di Bisceglie. A.M., S.E. Order, J.L. Klein, J.G. Waggoner, M.H. Sjogren, G. Kuo, M. Houghton, Q-L. Choo, J.H. Hoofnagle. 1991. The Role of Chronic Viral Hepatitis in Hepatocellular Carcinoma in the United States. *American Journal of Gastroenterology.* 86:335-338.

El-Serag, H.B., A.C. Mason. 1999. Rising Incidence of Hepatocellular Carcinoma in the United States. *New England Journal of Medicine.* 340:745-50.

Everson, Gregory T. 2000. Increasing Incidence and Pretransplantation Screening of Hepatocellular Carcinoma. *Liver Transplantation*. Vol. 6, No. 6, Suppl. 2 (Nov.):S2–S10.

Mazzaferro, V., E. Regalia, R. Doci, S. Andreola, A. Pulvirenti, F. Bozzetti, F. Montalto, M. Ammatuna, A. Morabito, L. Gennari. 1996. Liver Transplantation for the Treatment of Small Hepatocellular Carcinomas in Patients With Cirrhosis. *New England Journal of Medicine*. 334:693–699.

McMahon, B.J., L. Bulkow, A. Harpster, M. Snowball, A. Lanier, F. Sacco, E. Dunaway, J. Williams. 2000. Screening for Hepatocellular Carcinoma in Alaska Natives Infected With Chronic Hepatitis B: A 16-Year Population-Based Study. *Hepatology*. 32:842–846.

McMahon, B.J., T. London. 1991. Workshop on Screening for Hepatocellular Carcinoma. *Journal of the National Cancer Institute*. Vol. 83, No. 13 (July 3):916–919.

Penn, I. 1991. Hepatic Transplantation for Primary and Metastatic Cancers of the Liver. *Surgery*. 110:726–734.

Popper, H., D.A. Shafritz, J.H. Hoofnagle. 1987. Relation of the Hepatitis B Virus Carrier State to Hepatocellular Carcinoma. *Hepatology*. 7:764–772.

Takayama, T., M. Makuuchi, S. Hirohashi, M. Sakamoto, J. Yamamoto, K. Shimada, T. Kosuge, S. Okada, K. Takayasu, S. Yamasaki. 1998. Early Hepatocellular Carcinoma as an Entity with a High Rate of Surgical Cure. *Hepatology*. 28:1241–1246.

Williams, R., P. Rizzi. 1996. Treating Small Hepatocellular Carcinomas. *New England Journal of Medicine*. Vol. 334, No. 11: 728–729.

Wong, L.L., W.M. Limm, R. Severino, L.M. Wong. 2000. Improved Survival with Screening for Hepatocellular Carcinoma. *Liver Transplantation*. Vol. 6, No. 3 (May):320–325.

World Health Organization. *Prevention of Liver Cancer*. Technical Report Series 691. Geneva: WHO, 1983.

Yuen, M-F, C-C. Cheng, I.J. Lauder, S-K. Lam, C. G-C. Ooi, C-L. Lai. 2000. Early Detection of Hepatocellular Carcinoma Increases the Chance of Treatment: Hong Kong Experience. *Hepatology*. 31:330–335.

Chapter 11

Abramowicz, M., Ed. 1995. Drugs for AIDS and Associated Infections. *The Medical Letter on Drugs and Therapeutics*. Vol. 37 (Issue 959):87–94.

Benhamou, Y., M. Bochet, V. Thibault, V. DiMartino, E. Caumes, F. Bricaire, P. Opolon, C. Katlama, T. Poynard. 1999. Long-Term Incidence of Hepatitis B Virus Resistance to Lamivudine in Human Immunodeficiency Virus-Infected Patients. *Hepatology*. 30:1302–1306.

Benhamou, Y., C. Katlama, F. Lunel, A. Coutelier, E. Dohin, N. Hamm, R. Tubiana, S. Herson, T. Poynard, P. Opolon. 1996. Effects of Lamivudine on Replication of Hepatitis B Virus in HIV-Infected Men. *Annals of Internal Medicine*. 125:705–712.

Cacciola, I., T. Pollicino, G. Squadrito, G. Cerenzia, M.E. Orlando, G. Raimondo. 1999. Occult Hepatitis B Virus Infection in Patients with Chronic Hepatitis C Liver Disease. *New England Journal of Medicine*. 341:22–26.

Chang, C.J., Y.C. Ko, H.W. Liu. 2000. Serum Alanine Aminotransferase Levels in

Relation to Hepatitis B and C Virus Infections among Drug Abusers in an Area Hyperendemic for Hepatitis B. *Digestive Disease and Science*. 45:1949-1952.

Colin, J.F., D. Cazals-Hatem, M.A. Loriot, M. Martinot-Peignoux, B.N. Pham, A. Auperin, C. Degott, J..P. Benhamou, S. Erlinger, D.Valla, P. Marcellin. 1999. Influence of Human Immunodeficiency Virus Infection on Chronic Hepatitis B in Homosexual Men. *Hepatology*. 29:1306-1310.

DenBrinker, M., F.W.N.M. Witt, P.M.E. Wertheim-VanDillen, S. Jurriaans, J. Weel, R. Van Leeuwen, N.G. Pakkor, P. Reiss, S.A. Danner, G.J. Weverling, J.M.A. Lange. 2000. Hepatitis B and C Virus Co-Infection and the Risk for Hepatotoxicity of Highly Active Anti-retroviral Therapy in HIV-1 Infection. *AIDS*. 14:2895-2902.

Eyster, M.E., J.C. Sanders, M. Battegay, A.M. DiBisceglie. 1995. Suppression of Hepatitis C Virus (HCV) Replication by Hepatitis D virus (HDV) in HIV-Infected Hemophiliacs with Chronic Hepatitis B and C. *Digestive Disease and Science*. 40:1583-1588.

Farci, P., A. Mandas, A. Coiana, M.E. Lai, V. Desmet, P.VanEyken, Y. Gibo, L. Caruso, S. Scaccabarozzi, D. Criscuolo, J.C. Ryff, A. Balestrieri. 1994. Treatment of Chronic Hepatitis D with Interferon Alfa-2a. *New England Journal of Medicine*. 330:88-94.

Fong, T.L., A.M. DiBisceglie, J.G. Waggoner, S.M. Banks, J.H. Hoofnagle. 1991. The Significance of Antibody to Hepatitis C Virus in Patients with Chronic Hepatitis B. *Hepatology*. 14:64-67.

Gaeta, G.B., T. Stroffolini, M. Chiaramonte, T. Ascione, G. Stornaiuolo, S. Lobello, E. Sagnelli, M.R. Brunetto, M. Rizzetto. 2000. Chronic Hepatitis D: A Vanishing Disease? An Italian Multicenter Study. *Hepatology*. 32:824-827.

Kazemi-Shirazi, L., D. Petermann, C. Muller. 2000. Hepatitis B Virus DNA in Sera and Liver Tissue of HBsAg Negative Patients with Chronic Hepatitis C. *Journal of Hepatology*. 33:785-790.

Krogsgaard, K, B.O. Lindhardt, J.O. Nielsen, P. Andersson, P. Kryger, J. Aldershvile, J. Gerstoft, C. Pedersen. 1987. The Influence of HTLV-III Infection on the Natural History of Hepatitis B Virus Infection in Male Homosexual HBsAg Carriers. *Hepatology*. 7:37-41.

Lau, D.T.Y., E. Doo, Y. Park, D.E. Kleiner, P. Schmid, M.C. Kuhns, J.H. Hoofnagle. 1999. Lamivudine for Chronic Delta Hepatitis. *Hepatology*. 30:546-549.

Lau, D.T.Y., D.E. Kleiner, Y. Park, A.M. DiBisceglie, J.H. Hoofnagle. 1999. Resolution of Chronic Delta Hepatitis after 12 Years of Interferon Alfa Therapy. *Gastroenterology*. 117:1229-1233.

Manegold, C., C. Hannoun, A. Wywiol, M. Dietrich, S. Polywka, C.B. Chiwakata, S. Gunther. 2001. Reactivation of Hepatitis B Virus Replication Accompanied by Acute Hepatitis in Patients Receiving Highly Active Antiretroviral Therapy. *Clinical Infectious Diseases*. 2001. 32:144-148.

Remis, R.S., A. Dufour, M. Alary, J. Vincelette, J. Otis, B. Masse, B. Turmel, R. LeClerc, R. Parent, R. Lavoie. 2000. Association of Hepatitis B Virus Infection with Other Sexually Transmitted Infections in Homosexual Men. *American Journal of Public Health*. 90:1570-1574.

Rogers, A.S., J.C. Lindsey, D.C. Futterman, B. Zimmer, S.E. Abdalian, L.J. D'Angelo, The Pediatric AIDS Clinical Trials Group protocol 220 Team. 2000. Serologic

Examination of Hepatitis B Infection and Immunization in HIV-Positive Youth and Associated Risks. *AIDS Patient Care STDS.* 14 (12):651-657.

Rosina, F., P. Conoscitore, R. Cuppone, G. Rocca, A. Giulani, R. Cozzolongo, G. Niro, A. Smedile, G. Saracco, A. Andriulli, O.G. Manghisi, M. Rizzetto. 1999. Changing Pattern of Chronic Hepatitis D in Southern Europe. *Gastroenterology.* 117:161-166.

Sagnelli, E., N. Coppola, C. Scolastico, P. Filippini, T. Santantonio, T. Stroffolini, F. Piccinino. 2000. Virologic and Clinical Expressions of Reciprocal Inhibitory Effect of Hepatitis B, C, and Delta Viruses in Patients with Chronic Hepatitis. *Hepatology.* 32:1106-1110.

Selik, R.M., et al. April 2000. Increases in the Percentage with Liver Disease Among Deaths with HIV Infection. 10th International Symposium on Viral Hepatitis and Liver Disease; Atlanta, Georgia. (http://www.hivandhepatitis.com/hepb/bo4240002.html)

Wolters, L.M.M., A.B. Van Nunen, P. Honkoop, A.C.T.M. Vossen, H.G.M. Niesters, P.E. Zondervan, R.A. De Man. 2000. Lamivudine-High Dose Interferon Combination Therapy for Chronic Hepatitis B Patients Co-Infected with the Hepatitis D Virus. *Journal of Viral Hepatitis.* 7:428-434.

Chapter 12

ACOG Committee Opinion: Committee on Obstetrics: Maternal and Fetal Medicine, Number 78, January 1990. 1991. Guidelines for Hepatitis B Virus Screening and Vaccination During Pregnancy. *International Journal of Gynecology and Obstetrics.* 35:367-369.

Alter, M. 1996. Epidemiology and Disease Burden of Hepatitis B and C. *Antiviral Therapy.* 1 (suppl 3): 9-14

Barbera, C., F. Bortolotti, C. Crivellaro, A. Coscia, L. Zancan, P. Cadrobbi P, G. Nebbia, M.N. Pillan, L. Lepore, T. Parrella, G. Dastoli, M.R. Brunetto, F. Bonino. 1994. Recombinant Interferon-a Hastens the Rate of HBeAg Clearance in Children with Chronic Hepatitis B. *Hepatology.* 20:287-290.

Bortolotti, F. P. Cadrobbi, C. Crivellaro, M. Guido, M. Rugge, F. Noventa, R. Calzia, G. Realdi. 1990. Long-Term Outcome of Chronic Type B Hepatitis in Patients Who Acquire Hepatitis B Virus Infection in Childhood. *Gastroenterology.* 99:805-810.

Franks, A.L., C.J. Berg, M.A. Kane, B.B. Browne, K. Sikes, W.R. Elsea, A.H. Burton. 1989. Hepatitis B Virus Infection Among Children Born in the United States to Southeast Asian Refugees. *New England Journal of Medicine.* 31:321:1301-1305.

Friedt, M., P. Gerner, E. Lausch, H. Trubel, B. Zabel, S. Wirth. Mutations in the Basic Core Promoter and the Precore Region of Hepatitis B Virus and Their Selection in Children with Fulminant and Chronic Hepatitis B. *Hepatology.* 29:1252-1258.

Hershow, R.C., S.C. Hadler, M.A. Kane. 1987. Adoption of Children from Countries with Endemic Hepatitis B: Transmission, Risks, and Medical Issues. *Pediatric Infectious Diseases Journal.* 6:431-437.

Immunization Practices Advisory Committee (ACIP). 1991. Hepatitis B Virus: A

Comprehensive Strategy for Eliminating Transmission in the United States Through Universal Childhood Vaccination. *MMWR.* 40:1-19.

Jonas, Maureen M. 1998. Viral Hepatitis. *Pediatric Gastrointestinal Disease,* Vol. II, 2nd Edition. Walker, W. A., P. R. Durie, J. R. Hamilton, J. A. Walker-Smith, J. B. Watkins, eds. St. Louis: Mosby. 1028-1041.

Lok, A.S.F., C.L. Lai. 1988. A Longitudinal Follow-up of Asymptomatic Hepatitis B Surface Antigen Positive Chinese Children. *Hepatology.* 8:1130-113.

Lok, A.S.F., C.L. Lai, P.C. Wu, E.K.Y. Leung, T.S. Lam. 1987. Spontaneous Hepatitis e antigen to Antibody Seroconversion and Reversion in Chinese Patients with Chronic Hepatitis B Virus Infection. *Gastroenterology.* 92:1839-1843.

McMahon, B.J., W.L.M. Alward, D.B. Hall, W.L. Heyward, T.R. Bender, D.P. Francis, J.E. Maynard. 1985. Acute Hepatitis B Virus Infection: Relation of Age to the Clinical Expression of Disease and Subsequent Development of the Carrier State. *Journal of Infectious Diseases.* 151(4):599-603.

Narkewicz, M.R., D. Smith, A. Silverman, J. Vierling, R.J. Sokol. 1995. Clearance of Chronic Hepatitis B Virus Infection in Young Children After Alpha Interferon Treatment. *Journal of Pediatrics.* 127:815-8.

Pon, E.W., H. Ren, H. Margolis, Z. Zhao, G.C. Schatz, A. Diwan. 1993. Hepatitis B Virus Infection in Honolulu Students. *Pediatrics.* 92(4):574-578.

Ruiz-Moreno, M., M.J. Rua , J. Molina, G. Moraleda, A. Moreno, J. Garcia-Aguado, V. Carreno. 1991. Prospective Randomized Controlled Trial of Interferon-a in Children with Chronic Hepatitis B. *Hepatology.* 13:1035-1039.

Sokal, E.M., H.S. Conjeevaram, E.A. Roberts, F. Alvarez, E.M. Bern, P. Goyens, P. Rosenthal, A. Lachaux, M. Shelton, J. Sarles, J. Hoofnagle. 1998. Interferon Alfa Therapy for Chronic Hepatitis B in Children: A Multinational Randomized Controlled Trial. Gastroenterology. 114:988-995.

Thursz, M.R., D. Kwiatkowski, C.E.M. Allsopp, B.M. Greenwood, H.C. Thomas, A.V.S. Hill. 1995. Association Between an MHC Class II Allele and Clearance of Hepatitis B Virus in the Gambia. *New England Journal of Medicine.* 332:1065-1069.

Chapter 13

Andreone, P., C. Cursaro, A. Gramenzi, C. Zavaglia, I. Rezakovic, E. Altomare R. Severini, J.S. Franzone, O. Albano, G. Ideo, M. Bernardi, G. Gasbarrini. 1996. A Randomized Controlled Trial of Thymosin-alpha1 Versus Interferon Alfa Treatment in Patients with Hepatitis B e Antigen Antibody—and Hepatitis B Virus DNA—Positive Chronic Hepatitis B. *Hepatology.* 24:774-777.

Baptista, M., A. Kramvis, M.C. Kew. 1999. High Prevalence of 1762T 1764A Mutations in the Basic Core Promoter of Hepatitis B Virus Isolated from Black Africans with Hepatocellular Carcinoma Compared with Asymptomatic Carriers. *Hepatology.* 29:946-953.

Brown, J.L., W.F. Carman, H.C. Thomas. 1992. The Clinical Significance of Molecular Variation within the Hepatitis B Virus Genome. *Hepatology.* 15:144-148.

Carman, W.F., H.C. Thomas. 1992. Genetic Variation in Hepatitis B Virus. *Gastroenterology.* 102:711-719.

Davis, G.L. 1991. Treatment of Chronic Hepatitis B. *Hepatology.* 14:567-569.

Diepolder, H.M., G. Ries, M.C. Jung, H.J. Schlicht, J.T. Gerlach, N. Gruner, W.H. Caselmann, G.R. Pape. 1999. Differential Antigen-Processing Pathways of the Hepatitis B Virus e and Core Proteins. *Gastroenterology*. 116:650-657.

Doo, E., T.J. Liang. 2001. Molecular Anatomy and Pathophysiologic Implications of Drug Resistance in Hepatitis B Virus Infection. *Gastroenterology*. 120:1000-1008.

Heathcote, J., J. McHutchison, S. Lee, M. Tong, K. Benner, G. Minuk, T. Wright, J. Fikes, B. Livingston, A. Sette, R. Chestnut R, and the CY-1899 Vaccine Study Group. 1999. A Pilot Study of the CY-1899 T-Cell Vaccine in Subjects Chronically Infected with Hepatitis B Virus. *Hepatology*. 30:531-536.

Honda, M., S. Kaneko, H. Kawai, Y. Shirota, K. Kobayashi. 2001. Differential Gene Expression between Chronic Hepatitis B and C Hepatic Lesion. *Gastroenterology*. 120:955-966.

Hunt, C.M., J.M. McGill, M.I. Allen, L.D. Condreay. 2000. Clinical Relevance of Hepatitis B Viral Mutations. *Hepatology*. 31:1037-1044.

Inoue, K., M. Yoshiba, K. Sekiyama, H. Okamoto, M. Mayumi. 1998. Clinical and Molecular Virological Differences between Fulminant Hepatic Failures Following Acute and Chronic Infection with Hepatitis B Virus. *Journal of Medical Virology*. 55:35-41.

Kao, J.H., P.J. Chen, M.Y. Lai, D.S. Chen. 2000. Hepatitis B Genotypes Correlate with Clinical Outcomes in Patients with Chronic Hepatitis B. *Gastroenterology*. 118:554-559.

Malik, A.H., W.M. Lee. 2000. Chronic Hepatitis B Virus Infection: Treatment Strategies for the Next Millenium. *Annals of Internal Medicine*. 132:723-731.

Mason, A.L., L. Xu, L. Guo, M. Kuhns, R.P. Perrillo. 1998. Molecular Basis for Persistent Hepatitis B Virus Infection in the Liver after Clearance of Serum Hepatitis B Surface Antigen. *Hepatology*. 27:1736-1742.

Milich, D.R. 1999. Do T Cells "See" the Hepatitis B Core and e Antigens Differently? *Gastroenterology*. 116:765-768.

Mutchnick, M. G., H.D. Appelman, H.T. Chung, E. Aragona, T.P. Gupta, G.D. Cummings, J.G. Waggoner, J.H. Hoofnagle, D.A. Shafritz. 1991. Thymosin Treatment of Chronic Hepatitis B: A Placebo-controlled Pilot Trial. *Hepatology*. 14:409-415.

Perrillo, R.P. 2001. Acute Flares in Chronic Hepatitis B: The Natural and Unnatural History of an Immunologically Mediated Liver Disease. *Gastroenterology*. 120:1009-1022.

Pianko, S., J. McHutchison. 1999. Chronic Hepatitis B: New Therapies on the Horizon? *Lancet*. 354:1662-1663.

Torresi, J., S. Locarnini S. 2000. Antiviral Chemotherapy for the Treatment of Hepatitis B Virus Infection. *Gastroenterology*. 118:S83-S103.

Index